THE OFFICIAL PATIENT'S SOURCEBOOK

on

IMMUNE THROMBOCYTOPENIC PURPURA

JAMES N. PARKER, M.D.
AND PHILIP M. PARKER, PH.D., EDITORS

ICON Health Publications
ICON Group International, Inc.
4370 La Jolla Village Drive, 4th Floor
San Diego, CA 92122 USA

Printed in the United States of America.

Last digit indicates print number: 10 9 8 7 6 4 5 3 2 1

Publisher, Health Care: Tiffany LaRochelle
Editor(s): James Parker, M.D., Philip Parker, Ph.D.

Publisher's note: The ideas, procedures, and suggestions contained in this book are not intended as a substitute for consultation with your physician. All matters regarding your health require medical supervision. As new medical or scientific information becomes available from academic and clinical research, recommended treatments and drug therapies may undergo changes. The authors, editors, and publisher have attempted to make the information in this book up to date and accurate in accord with accepted standards at the time of publication. The authors, editors, and publisher are not responsible for errors or omissions or for consequences from application of the book, and make no warranty, expressed or implied, in regard to the contents of this book. Any practice described in this book should be applied by the reader in accordance with professional standards of care used in regard to the unique circumstances that may apply in each situation, in close consultation with a qualified physician. The reader is advised to always check product information (package inserts) for changes and new information regarding dose and contraindications before taking any drug or pharmacological product. Caution is especially urged when using new or infrequently ordered drugs, herbal remedies, vitamins and supplements, alternative therapies, complementary therapies and medicines, and integrative medical treatments.

Cataloging-in-Publication Data

Parker, James N., 1961-
Parker, Philip M., 1960-

The Official Patient's Sourcebook on Immune Thrombocytopenic Purpura: A Revised and Updated Directory for the Internet Age/James N. Parker and Philip M. Parker, editors
            p.   cm.
Includes bibliographical references, glossary and index.
ISBN: 0-597-83152-1
1. Immune Thrombocytopenic Purpura-Popular works.   I. Title.

Disclaimer

This publication is not intended to be used for the diagnosis or treatment of a health problem or as a substitute for consultation with licensed medical professionals. It is sold with the understanding that the publisher, editors, and authors are not engaging in the rendering of medical, psychological, financial, legal, or other professional services.

References to any entity, product, service, or source of information that may be contained in this publication should not be considered an endorsement, either direct or implied, by the publisher, editors or authors. ICON Group International, Inc., the editors, or the authors are not responsible for the content of any Web pages nor publications referenced in this publication.

Copyright Notice

Dedication

To the healthcare professionals dedicating their time and efforts to the study of immune thrombocytopenic purpura.

Acknowledgements

The collective knowledge generated from academic and applied research summarized in various references has been critical in the creation of this sourcebook which is best viewed as a comprehensive compilation and collection of information prepared by various official agencies which directly or indirectly are dedicated to immune thrombocytopenic purpura. All of the *Official Patient's Sourcebooks* draw from various agencies and institutions associated with the United States Department of Health and Human Services, and in particular, the Office of the Secretary of Health and Human Services (OS), the Administration for Children and Families (ACF), the Administration on Aging (AOA), the Agency for Healthcare Research and Quality (AHRQ), the Agency for Toxic Substances and Disease Registry (ATSDR), the Centers for Disease Control and Prevention (CDC), the Food and Drug Administration (FDA), the Healthcare Financing Administration (HCFA), the Health Resources and Services Administration (HRSA), the Indian Health Service (IHS), the institutions of the National Institutes of Health (NIH), the Program Support Center (PSC), and the Substance Abuse and Mental Health Services Administration (SAMHSA). In addition to these sources, information gathered from the National Library of Medicine, the United States Patent Office, the European Union, and their related organizations has been invaluable in the creation of this sourcebook. Some of the work represented was financially supported by the Research and Development Committee at INSEAD. This support is gratefully acknowledged. Finally, special thanks are owed to Tiffany LaRochelle for her excellent editorial support.

About the Editors

James N. Parker, M.D.

Dr. James N. Parker received his Bachelor of Science degree in Psychobiology from the University of California, Riverside and his M.D. from the University of California, San Diego. In addition to authoring numerous research publications, he has lectured at various academic institutions. Dr. Parker is the medical editor for the *Official Patient's Sourcebook* series published by ICON Health Publications.

Philip M. Parker, Ph.D.

Philip M. Parker is the Eli Lilly Chair Professor of Innovation, Business and Society at INSEAD (Fontainebleau, France and Singapore). Dr. Parker has also been Professor at the University of California, San Diego and has taught courses at Harvard University, the Hong Kong University of Science and Technology, the Massachusetts Institute of Technology, Stanford University, and UCLA. Dr. Parker is the associate editor for the *Official Patient's Sourcebook* series published by ICON Health Publications.

About ICON Health Publications

In addition to hemophilia, *Official Patient's Sourcebooks* are available for the following related topics:

- The Official Patient's Sourcebook on Hemophilia
- The Official Patient's Sourcebook on Raynaud
- The Official Patient's Sourcebook on Sickle Cell Anemia

To discover more about ICON Health Publications, simply check with your preferred online booksellers, including Barnes & Noble.com and Amazon.com which currently carry all of our titles. Or, feel free to contact us directly for bulk purchases or institutional discounts:

ICON Group International, Inc.
4370 La Jolla Village Drive, Fourth Floor
San Diego, CA 92122 USA
Fax: 858-546-4341
Web site: **www.icongrouponline.com/health**

Table of Contents

INTRODUCTION

Overview

Dr. C. Everett Koop, former U.S. Surgeon General, once said, "The best prescription is knowledge."[1] The Agency for Healthcare Research and Quality (AHRQ) of the National Institutes of Health (NIH) echoes this view and recommends that every patient incorporate education into the treatment process. According to the AHRQ:

> Finding out more about your condition is a good place to start. By contacting groups that support your condition, visiting your local library, and searching on the Internet, you can find good information to help guide your treatment decisions. Some information may be hard to find — especially if you don't know where to look.[2]

As the AHRQ mentions, finding the right information is not an obvious task. Though many physicians and public officials had thought that the emergence of the Internet would do much to assist patients in obtaining reliable information, in March 2001 the National Institutes of Health issued the following warning:

> The number of Web sites offering health-related resources grows every day. Many sites provide valuable information, while others may have information that is unreliable or misleading.[3]

---

[1] Quotation from **http://www.drkoop.com**.

[2] The Agency for Healthcare Research and Quality (AHRQ):
http://www.ahcpr.gov/consumer/diaginfo.htm.

[3] From the NIH, National Cancer Institute (NCI):
http://cancertrials.nci.nih.gov/beyond/evaluating.html.

Since the late 1990s, physicians have seen a general increase in patient Internet usage rates. Patients frequently enter their doctor's offices with printed Web pages of home remedies in the guise of latest medical research. This scenario is so common that doctors often spend more time dispelling misleading information than guiding patients through sound therapies. *The Official Patient's Sourcebook on Immune Thrombocytopenic Purpura* has been created for patients who have decided to make education and research an integral part of the treatment process. The pages that follow will tell you where and how to look for information covering virtually all topics related to immune thrombocytopenic purpura, from the essentials to the most advanced areas of research.

The title of this book includes the word "official." This reflects the fact that the sourcebook draws from public, academic, government, and peer-reviewed research. Selected readings from various agencies are reproduced to give you some of the latest official information available to date on immune thrombocytopenic purpura.

Given patients' increasing sophistication in using the Internet, abundant references to reliable Internet-based resources are provided throughout this sourcebook. Where possible, guidance is provided on how to obtain free-of-charge, primary research results as well as more detailed information via the Internet. E-book and electronic versions of this sourcebook are fully interactive with each of the Internet sites mentioned (clicking on a hyperlink automatically opens your browser to the site indicated). Hard copy users of this sourcebook can type cited Web addresses directly into their browsers to obtain access to the corresponding sites. Since we are working with ICON Health Publications, hard copy *Sourcebooks* are frequently updated and printed on demand to ensure that the information provided is current.

In addition to extensive references accessible via the Internet, every chapter presents a "Vocabulary Builder." Many health guides offer glossaries of technical or uncommon terms in an appendix. In editing this sourcebook, we have decided to place a smaller glossary within each chapter that covers terms used in that chapter. Given the technical nature of some chapters, you may need to revisit many sections. Building one's vocabulary of medical terms in such a gradual manner has been shown to improve the learning process.

We must emphasize that no sourcebook on immune thrombocytopenic purpura should affirm that a specific diagnostic procedure or treatment discussed in a research study, patent, or doctoral dissertation is "correct" or your best option. This sourcebook is no exception. Each patient is unique.

Deciding on appropriate options is always up to the patient in consultation with their physician and healthcare providers.

Organization

This sourcebook is organized into three parts. Part I explores basic techniques to researching immune thrombocytopenic purpura (e.g. finding guidelines on diagnosis, treatments, and prognosis), followed by a number of topics, including information on how to get in touch with organizations, associations, or other patient networks dedicated to immune thrombocytopenic purpura. It also gives you sources of information that can help you find a doctor in your local area specializing in treating immune thrombocytopenic purpura. Collectively, the material presented in Part I is a complete primer on basic research topics for patients with immune thrombocytopenic purpura.

Part II moves on to advanced research dedicated to immune thrombocytopenic purpura. Part II is intended for those willing to invest many hours of hard work and study. It is here that we direct you to the latest scientific and applied research on immune thrombocytopenic purpura. When possible, contact names, links via the Internet, and summaries are provided. It is in Part II where the vocabulary process becomes important as authors publishing advanced research frequently use highly specialized language. In general, every attempt is made to recommend "free-to-use" options.

Part III provides appendices of useful background reading for all patients with immune thrombocytopenic purpura or related disorders. The appendices are dedicated to more pragmatic issues faced by many patients with immune thrombocytopenic purpura. Accessing materials via medical libraries may be the only option for some readers, so a guide is provided for finding local medical libraries which are open to the public. Part III, therefore, focuses on advice that goes beyond the biological and scientific issues facing patients with immune thrombocytopenic purpura.

Scope

While this sourcebook covers immune thrombocytopenic purpura, your doctor, research publications, and specialists may refer to your condition using a variety of terms. Therefore, you should understand that immune thrombocytopenic purpura is often considered a synonym or a condition closely related to the following:

- Autoimmune Thrombocytopenic Purpura
- Idiopathic Thrombocytopenic Purpura
- Postinfectious Thrombocytopenia
- Purpura Hemorrhagica Itp
- Werlhof Disease
- Werlhof's Disease

In addition to synonyms and related conditions, physicians may refer to immune thrombocytopenic purpura using certain coding systems. The International Classification of Diseases, 9th Revision, Clinical Modification (ICD-9-CM) is the most commonly used system of classification for the world's illnesses. Your physician may use this coding system as an administrative or tracking tool. The following dassification is commonly used for immune thrombocytopenic purpura:[4]

- 287.3 idiopathic thrombocy-topenic purpura (itp)
- 287.3 primary thrombocytopenia

For the purposes of this sourcebook, we have attempted to be as inclusive as possible, looking for official information for all of the synonyms relevant to immune thrombocytopenic purpura. You may find it useful to refer to synonyms when accessing databases or interacting with healthcare professionals and medical librarians.

Moving Forward

Since the 1980s, the world has seen a proliferation of healthcare guides covering most illnesses. Some are written by patients or their family members. These generally take a layperson's approach to understanding and coping with an illness or disorder. They can be uplifting, encouraging, and highly supportive. Other guides are authored by physicians or other

---

[4] This list is based on the official version of the World Health Organization's 9th Revision, International Classification of Diseases (ICD-9). According to the National Technical Information Service, "ICD-9CM extensions, interpretations, modifications, addenda, or errata other than those approved by the U.S. Public Health Service and the Health Care Financing Administration are not to be considered official and should not be utilized. Continuous maintenance of the ICD-9-CM is the responsibility of the federal government."

healthcare providers who have a more clinical outlook. Each of these two styles of guide has its purpose and can be quite useful.

As editors, we have chosen a third route. We have chosen to expose you to as many sources of official and peer-reviewed information as practical, for the purpose of educating you about basic and advanced knowledge as recognized by medical science today. You can think of this sourcebook as your personal Internet age reference librarian.

Why "Internet age"? All too often, patients diagnosed with immune thrombocytopenic purpura will log on to the Internet, type words into a search engine, and receive several Web site listings which are mostly irrelevant or redundant. These patients are left to wonder where the relevant information is, and how to obtain it. Since only the smallest fraction of information dealing with immune thrombocytopenic purpura is even indexed in search engines, a non-systematic approach often leads to frustration and disappointment. With this sourcebook, we hope to direct you to the information you need that you would not likely find using popular Web directories. Beyond Web listings, in many cases we will reproduce brief summaries or abstracts of available reference materials. These abstracts often contain distilled information on topics of discussion.

Before beginning your search for information, it is important for you to realize that immune thrombocytopenic purpura is considered a relatively uncommon condition. Because of this, far less research is conducted on immune thrombocytopenic purpura compared to other health problems afflicting larger populations, like breast cancer or heart disease. Nevertheless, this sourcebook will prove useful for two reasons. First, if more information does become available on immune thrombocytopenic purpura, the sources given in this book will be the most likely to report or make such information available. Second, some will find it important to know about patient support, symptom management, or diagnostic procedures that may be relevant to both immune thrombocytopenic purpura and other conditions. By using the sources listed in the following chapters, self-directed research can be conducted on broader topics that are related to immune thrombocytopenic purpura but not readily uncovered using general Internet search engines (e.g. **www.google.com** or **www.yahoo.com**). In this way, we have designed this sourcebook to complement these general search engines that can provide useful information and access to online patient support groups.[5]

_____

[5] For example, one can simply go to **www.google.com,** or other general search engines (e.g. **www.yahoo.com**, **www.aol.com**, **www.msn.com**) and type in "diseasex support group" to find any active online support groups dedicated to diseasex.

While we focus on the more scientific aspects of immune thrombocytopenic purpura, there is, of course, the emotional side to consider. Later in the sourcebook, we provide a chapter dedicated to helping you find peer groups and associations that can provide additional support beyond research produced by medical science. We hope that the choices we have made give you the most options available in moving forward. In this way, we wish you the best in your efforts to incorporate this educational approach into your treatment plan.

The Editors

PART I: THE ESSENTIALS

ABOUT PART I

Part I has been edited to give you access to what we feel are "the essentials" on immune thrombocytopenic purpura. The essentials of a disease typically include the definition or description of the disease, a discussion of who it affects, the signs or symptoms associated with the disease, tests or diagnostic procedures that might be specific to the disease, and treatments for the disease. Your doctor or healthcare provider may have already explained the essentials of immune thrombocytopenic purpura to you or even given you a pamphlet or brochure describing immune thrombocytopenic purpura. Now you are searching for more in-depth information. As editors, we have decided, nevertheless, to include a discussion on where to find essential information that can complement what your doctor has already told you. In this section we recommend a process, not a particular Web site or reference book. The process ensures that, as you search the Web, you gain background information in such a way as to maximize your understanding.

Chapter 1. The Essentials on Immune Thrombocytopenic Purpura: Guidelines

Overview

Official agencies, as well as federally-funded institutions supported by national grants, frequently publish a variety of guidelines on immune thrombocytopenic purpura. These are typically called "Fact Sheets" or "Guidelines." They can take the form of a brochure, information kit, pamphlet, or flyer. Often they are only a few pages in length. The great advantage of guidelines over other sources is that they are often written with the patient in mind. Since new guidelines on immune thrombocytopenic purpura can appear at any moment and be published by a number of sources, the best approach to finding guidelines is to systematically scan the Internet-based services that post them.

The National Institutes of Health (NIH)[6]

The National Institutes of Health (NIH) is the first place to search for relatively current patient guidelines and fact sheets on immune thrombocytopenic purpura. Originally founded in 1887, the NIH is one of the world's foremost medical research centers and the federal focal point for medical research in the United States. At any given time, the NIH supports some 35,000 research grants at universities, medical schools, and other research and training institutions, both nationally and internationally. The rosters of those who have conducted research or who have received NIH support over the years include the world's most illustrious scientists and

---

[6] Adapted from the NIH: http://www.nih.gov/about/NIHoverview.html.

physicians. Among them are 97 scientists who have won the Nobel Prize for achievement in medicine.

There is no guarantee that any one Institute will have a guideline on a specific disease, though the National Institutes of Health collectively publish over 600 guidelines for both common and rare diseases. The best way to access NIH guidelines is via the Internet. Although the NIH is organized into many different Institutes and Offices, the following is a list of key Web sites where you are most likely to find NIH clinical guidelines and publications dealing with immune thrombocytopenic purpura and associated conditions:

- Office of the Director (OD); guidelines consolidated across agencies available at **http://www.nih.gov/health/consumer/conkey.htm**

- National Library of Medicine (NLM); extensive encyclopedia (A.D.A.M., Inc.) with guidelines available at **http://www.nlm.nih.gov/medlineplus/healthtopics.html**

- National Heart, Lung, and Blood Institute (NHLBI); guidelines at **http://www.nhlbi.nih.gov/guidelines/index.htm**

Among these, the National Heart, Lung, and Blood Institute (NHLBI) is particularly noteworthy. The NHLBI provides leadership for a national program in diseases of the heart, blood vessels, lung, and blood; blood resources; and sleep disorders.[7] Since October 1997, the NHLBI has also had administrative responsibility for the NIH Woman's Health Initiative. The Institute plans, conducts, fosters, and supports an integrated and coordinated program of basic research, clinical investigations and trials, observational studies, and demonstration and education projects. Research is related to the causes, prevention, diagnosis, and treatment of heart, blood vessel, lung, and blood diseases; and sleep disorders. The NHLBI plans and directs research in development and evaluation of interventions and devices related to prevention, treatment, and rehabilitation of patients suffering from such diseases and disorders. It also supports research on clinical use of blood and all aspects of the management of blood resources. Research is conducted in the Institute's own laboratories and by scientific institutions and individuals supported by research grants and contracts. For health professionals and the public, the NHLBI conducts educational activities, including development and dissemination of materials in the above areas, with an emphasis on prevention.

---

[7] This paragraph has been adapted from the NHLBI: **http://www.nhlbi.nih.gov/about/org/mission.htm**. "Adapted" signifies that a passage is reproduced exactly or slightly edited for this book.

Within the NHLBI, the Division of Blood Diseases and Resources (DBDR) plans, directs, and evaluates the Institute's programs in hematology, hematologic diseases (except malignancies of the blood), and immunologic and other disorders of white blood cells, transfusion medicine, blood resources, and marrow and stem cell transplantation.[8] These programs include basic research, prevention, applied research and development, clinical trials, education, demonstration, and control activities. The Division monitors current activities and national needs and seeks to develop and support research into the causes, prevention, diagnosis, and treatment of diseases of the blood. Research on the use of blood and blood components in the treatment and prevention of diseases and the management of the nation's blood resources and transplantable tissue are also supported. A variety of support mechanisms are utilized, including research grants, contracts, cooperative agreements, centers, grants, career development awards, fellowships, and research training grants. Two programs comprise the DBDR: the Blood Diseases Program and the Blood Resources Program. The following patient guideline was recently published by the NHLBI and the DBDR on immune thrombocytopenic purpura.

What Is Immune Thrombocytopenic Purpura?[9]

Immune Thrombocytopenic Purpura (ITP) is a disorder of the blood. Immune refers to the immune system's involvement in this disorder. Antibodies, part of the body's immunologic defense against infection, attach to blood platelet, cells that help stop bleeding, and cause their destruction. Thrombocytopenia refers to decrease in blood platelet. Purpura refers to the purplish- looking areas of the skin and mucous membranes (such as the lining of the mouth) where bleeding has occurred as a result of decreased platelet.

Some cases of ITP are caused by drugs, and others are associated with infection, pregnancy, or immune disorders such as systemic lupus erythematosus. About half of all cases are classified as "idiopathic," meaning the cause is unknown.

---

[8] This paragraph has been adapted from the DBDR:
http://www.nhlbi.nih.gov/about/dbdr/index.htm . For more information, contact: Division of Blood Diseases and Resources; The National Heart, Lung and Blood Institute; ATTN: Web Site Inquiries; Two Rockledge Center, Suite 10138; 6701 Rockledge Dr., MSC 7950; Bethesda, Maryland 20892-7950.
[9] Adapted from the National Heart, Lung, and Blood Institute:
http://www.nhlbi.nih.gov/health/public/blood/other/tcp.txt.

What Are the Symptoms of ITP?

The main symptom is bleeding which can include bruising ("ecchymosis") and tiny red dots on the skin or mucous membranes ("petechiae"). In some instances bleeding from the nose, gums, digestive or urinary tracts may also occur. Rarely, bleeding within the brain occurs.

How Is ITP Diagnosed?

The physician will take a medical history and perform a thorough physical examination. A careful review of medications the patient is taking is important because some drugs can be associated with thrombocytopenia. A complete blood count will be done. A low platelet count will establish thrombocytopenia as the cause of purpura. Often the next procedure is a bone marrow examination to verify that there are adequate platelet-forming cells (megakaryocyte) in the marrow and to rule out other diseases such as metastatic cancer (cancer that has spread to the bone marrow) and leukemia cancer of the blood cells themselves). Another blood sample may be drawn to check for other conditions sometimes associated with thrombocytopenia such as lupus and infection.

Acute and Chronic Form of Thrombocytopenic Purpura

Acute (temporary) thrombocytopenic purpura is most commonly seen in young children. Boys and girls are equally affected. Symptoms often, but do not necessarily, follow a viral infection. About 85 percent of children recover within 1 year and the problem doesn't return.

Thrombocytopenic purpura is considered chronic when it has lasted more than 6 months. The onset of illness may be at any age. Adults more often have the chronic disorder and females are affected two to three times more than males. The onset of illness may be at any age.

How Is ITP Treated?

If the doctor thinks a drug is the cause of the thrombocytopenia, standard treatment involves discontinuing the drug's use. Infection, if present, is treated vigorously since control of the infection may result in a return of the platelet count to normal.

The treatment of idiopathic thrombocytopenic purpura is determined by the severity of the symptoms. In some cases, no therapy is needed. In most cases, drugs that alter the immune system's attack on the platelet are prescribed. These include corticosteroids (i.e., prednisone) and/or intravenous infusions of immune globulin. Another treatment that usually results in an increased number of platelet is removal of the spleen, the organ that destroys antibody-coated platelet. Other drugs such as vincristine, azathioprine (Imuran), Danazol, cyclophosphamide, and cyclosporine are prescribed for patients only in the severe case where other treatments have not shown benefit since these drugs have potentially harmful side effects.

Excepts in certain situation (e.g., internal bleeding and preparation for surgery), platelet transfusion usually are not beneficial and, therefore, are seldom performed. Because all therapies can have risks, it is important that overtreatment (treatment based solely on platelet counts and not on symptoms) be avoided. In some instances lifestyle adjustments may be helpful for prevention of bleeding due to injury. These would include use of protective gear such as helmets and avoidance of contact sports in symptomatic patients or when platelet counts are less than 50,000. Otherwise, patients usually can carry on normal activities, but final decisions about activity should be made in consultation with the patient's hematologist.

Where Can I Obtain Further Information on ITP?

Blood specialists (hematologist) are experts in the diagnosis and treatment of these disorders. These doctors practice in most mid-and large-size cities. A majority of medical centers have hematology divisions in their medicine or pediatrics departments, and patients who need evaluation, treatment, or information can often be referred there.

Additional information can be obtained from:

The National Organization for Rare Disorders
P.O. Box 8923
New Fairfield, Connecticut 06812
Telephone: (203) 746-6518

More Guideline Sources

The guideline above on immune thrombocytopenic purpura is only one example of the kind of material that you can find online and free of charge. The remainder of this chapter will direct you to other sources which either publish or can help you find additional guidelines on topics related to immune thrombocytopenic purpura. Many of the guidelines listed below address topics that may be of particular relevance to your specific situation or of special interest to only some patients with immune thrombocytopenic purpura. Due to space limitations these sources are listed in a concise manner. Do not hesitate to consult the following sources by either using the Internet hyperlink provided, or, in cases where the contact information is provided, contacting the publisher or author directly.

Topic Pages: MEDLINEplus

For patients wishing to go beyond guidelines published by specific Institutes of the NIH, the National Library of Medicine has created a vast and patient-oriented healthcare information portal called MEDLINEplus. Within this Internet-based system are "health topic pages." You can think of a health topic page as a guide to patient guides. To access this system, log on to **http://www.nlm.nih.gov/medlineplus/healthtopics.html**. From there you can either search using the alphabetical index or browse by broad topic areas.

If you do not find topics of interest when browsing health topic pages, then you can choose to use the advanced search utility of MEDLINEplus at **http://www.nlm.nih.gov/medlineplus/advancedsearch.html**. This utility is similar to the NIH Search Utility, with the exception that it only includes material linked within the MEDLINEplus system (mostly patient-oriented information). It also has the disadvantage of generating unstructured results. We recommend, therefore, that you use this method only if you have a very targeted search.

The National Guideline Clearinghouse™

The National Guideline Clearinghouse™ offers hundreds of evidence-based clinical practice guidelines published in the United States and other countries. You can search their site located at **http://www.guideline.gov** by using the keyword "immune thrombocytopenic purpura" or synonyms. The following was recently posted:

- **Idiopathic thrombocytopenic purpura: a practice guideline developed by explicit methods for the American Society of Hematology.**

  Source: American Society of Hematology.; 1996 January 25 (reviewed 2001); 91 pages

  http://www.guideline.gov/FRAMESETS/guideline_fs.asp?guideline=00 1148&sSearch_string=immune+thrombocytopenic+purpura

Healthfinder™

Healthfinder™ is an additional source sponsored by the U.S. Department of Health and Human Services which offers links to hundreds of other sites that contain healthcare information. This Web site is located at **http://www.healthfinder.gov**. Again, keyword searches can be used to find guidelines. The following was recently found in this database:

- **Facts About Immune Thrombocytopenic Purpura**

  Summary: Answers your questions about ITP, a disorder of the blood caused, in some cases by drugs, and in others is associated with infection, pregnancy, or immune disorders such as systemic lupus

  Source: National Heart, Lung, and Blood Institute, National Institutes of Health

  http://www.healthfinder.gov/scripts/recordpass.asp?RecordType=0&R ecordID=93

The NIH Search Utility

After browsing the references listed at the beginning of this chapter, you may want to explore the NIH Search Utility. This allows you to search for documents on over 100 selected Web sites that comprise the NIH-WEB-SPACE. Each of these servers is "crawled" and indexed on an ongoing basis. Your search will produce a list of various documents, all of which will relate in some way to immune thrombocytopenic purpura. The drawbacks of this approach are that the information is not organized by theme and that the references are often a mix of information for professionals and patients. Nevertheless, a large number of the listed Web sites provide useful background information. We can only recommend this route, therefore, for relatively rare or specific disorders, or when using highly targeted searches. To use the NIH search utility, visit the following Web page: **http://search.nih.gov/index.html**.

Additional Web Sources

A number of Web sites that often link to government sites are available to the public. These can also point you in the direction of essential information. The following is a representative sample:

- AOL: **http://search.aol.com/cat.adp?id=168&layer=&from=subcats**

- drkoop.com®: **http://www.drkoop.com/conditions/ency/index.html**

- Family Village: **http://www.familyvillage.wisc.edu/specific.htm**

- Google: **http://directory.google.com/Top/Health/Conditions_and_Diseases/**

- Med Help International: **http://www.medhelp.org/HealthTopics/A.html**

- Open Directory Project: **http://dmoz.org/Health/Conditions_and_Diseases/**

- Yahoo.com: **http://dir.yahoo.com/Health/Diseases_and_Conditions/**

- WebMD®Health: **http://my.webmd.com/health_topics**

Vocabulary Builder

The material in this chapter may have contained a number of unfamiliar words. The following Vocabulary Builder introduces you to terms used in this chapter that have not been covered in the previous chapter:

Antibody: An immunoglobulin molecule that has a specific amino acid sequence by virtue of which it interacts only with the antigen that induced its synthesis in cells of the lymphoid series (especially plasma cells), or with antigen closely related to it. Antibodies are classified according to their ode of action as agglutinins, bacteriolysins, haemolysins, opsonins, precipitins, etc. [EU]

Cell: Basic subunit of every living organism; the simplest unit that can exist as an independent living system. [NIH]

Chronic: Of long duration; frequently recurring. [NIH]

Corticosteroids: Drugs that mimic the action of a group of hormones produced by adrenal glands; they are anti-inflammatory and act as bronchodilators. [NIH]

Cyclophosphamide: Precursor of an alkylating nitrogen mustard antineoplastic and immunosuppressive agent that must be activated in the liver to form the active aldophosphamide. It is used in the treatment of lymphomas, leukemias, etc. Its side effect, alopecia, has been made use of in defleecing sheep. Cyclophosphamide may also cause sterility, birth defects, mutations, and cancer. [NIH]

Danazol: A synthetic steroid with antigonadotropic and anti-estrogenic activities that acts as an anterior pituitary suppressant by inhibiting the pituitary output of gonadotropins. It possesses some androgenic properties. Danazol has been used in the treatment of endometriosis and some benign breast disorders. [NIH]

Ecchymosis: A small haemorrhagic spot, larger than a petechia, in the skin or mucous membrane forming a nonelevated, rounded or irregular, blue or purplish patch. [EU]

Hematology: A subspecialty of internal medicine concerned with morphology, physiology, and pathology of the blood and blood-forming tissues. [NIH]

Idiopathic: Results from an unknown cause. [NIH]

Infusion: The therapeutic introduction of a fluid other than blood, as saline solution, solution, into a vein. [EU]

Intravenous: Within a vein or veins. [EU]

Lupus: A form of cutaneous tuberculosis. It is seen predominantly in women and typically involves the nasal, buccal, and conjunctival mucosa. [NIH]

Membrane: Thin, flexible film of proteins and lipids that encloses the contents of a cell; it controls the substances that go into and come out of the cell. Also, a thin layer of tissue that covers the surface or lines the cavity of an organ. [NIH]

Pediatrics: A medical specialty concerned with maintaining health and providing medical care to children from birth to adolescence. [NIH]

Prednisone: A synthetic anti-inflammatory glucocorticoid derived from cortisone. It is biologically inert and converted to prednisolone in the liver. [NIH]

Purpura: Purplish or brownish red discoloration, easily visible through the epidermis, caused by hemorrhage into the tissues. [NIH]

Symptomatic: 1. pertaining to or of the nature of a symptom. 2. indicative (of a particular disease or disorder). 3. exhibiting the symptoms of a particular disease but having a different cause. 4. directed at the allying of symptoms, as symptomatic treatment. [EU]

Systemic: Relating to a process that affects the body generally; in this instance, the way in which blood is supplied through the aorta to all body organs except the lungs. [NIH]

Thrombocytopenia: Decrease in the number of blood platelets. [EU]

Transfusion: The introduction of whole blood or blood component directly into the blood stream. [EU]

Transplantation: The grafting of tissues taken from the patient's own body or from another. [EU]

Urinary: Pertaining to the urine; containing or secreting urine. [EU]

Viral: Pertaining to, caused by, or of the nature of virus. [EU]

CHAPTER 2. SEEKING GUIDANCE

Overview

Some patients are comforted by the knowledge that a number of organizations dedicate their resources to helping people with immune thrombocytopenic purpura. These associations can become invaluable sources of information and advice. Many associations offer aftercare support, financial assistance, and other important services. Furthermore, healthcare research has shown that support groups often help people to better cope with their conditions.[10] In addition to support groups, your physician can be a valuable source of guidance and support. Therefore, finding a physician that can work with your unique situation is a very important aspect of your care.

In this chapter, we direct you to resources that can help you find patient organizations and medical specialists. We begin by describing how to find associations and peer groups that can help you better understand and cope with immune thrombocytopenic purpura. The chapter ends with a discussion on how to find a doctor that is right for you.

Associations and Immune Thrombocytopenic Purpura

As mentioned by the Agency for Healthcare Research and Quality, sometimes the emotional side of an illness can be as taxing as the physical side.[11] You may have fears or feel overwhelmed by your situation. Everyone has different ways of dealing with disease or physical injury. Your attitude,

---

[10] Churches, synagogues, and other houses of worship might also have groups that can offer you the social support you need.

[11] This section has been adapted from **http://www.ahcpr.gov/consumer/diaginf5.htm**.

your expectations, and how well you cope with your condition can all influence your well-being. This is true for both minor conditions and serious illnesses. For example, a study on female breast cancer survivors revealed that women who participated in support groups lived longer and experienced better quality of life when compared with women who did not participate. In the support group, women learned coping skills and had the opportunity to share their feelings with other women in the same situation.

In addition to associations or groups that your doctor might recommend, we suggest that you consider the following list (if there is a fee for an association, you may want to check with your insurance provider to find out if the cost will be covered):

- **Children's Blood Foundation**

  Address: Children's Blood Foundation 333 East 38th Street, Room 830, New York, NY 10016-2745

  Telephone: (212) 297-4336 Toll-free: (800) 487-701

  Fax: (212) 297-4340

  Email: cbf@nyh.med.cornell.ed

  Background: The Children's Blood Foundation (CBF) is a nonprofit organization dedicated to promoting and/or supporting research, medical training of physicians, and care of children with leukemia, thalassemia, hemophilia, anemia, cancer, immune disorders, and AIDS. Established in 1952, the CBF has the largest hemophilia center in the New York area and the largest thalassemia center in North America, receiving more than 5,000 patient visits every year. All affected children are served, regardless of the family's ability to pay. Educational materials include a self-titled brochure, a regular newsletter entitled 'The Key to Life for a Child,' and a booklet entitled 'What's It Called Again? - Answers to the Most Commonly Asked Questions About Idiopathic Thrombocytopenic Purpura (ITP) In Children.' CBF has support groups, offers networking services, and engages in educational activities.

  Relevant area(s) of interest: Idiopathic Thrombocytopenic Purpura

- **ITP Association**

  Address: ITP Association 45/8 Avraham Keren Street, Kfar Saba, 44208, Israel

  Telephone: 972-9-7657950

  Fax: 972-9-7410784 E-

  Background: The ITP (Idiopathic Thrombocytopenic Purpura) Association was established in 1997 in Israel as a support group for individuals with ITP, a condition characterized by deficiency of circulating blood platelets resulting in bleeding into the skin and other organs. The Association is committed to providing its members with current information concerning ITP research and its treatment, conducting periodic meetings with guest speakers from all medical and para-medical fields, promoting and supporting ITP research programs all over the world, and continually working to locate ITP specialists who will support such research. The ITP Association exchanges information with the ITP Society in New York and the Association in England; supports the Hebrew language in written and spoken forms; supports the French language in written form only; and distributes educational materials to its members. Such materials include leaflets and a regular newsletter. The Association welcomes all those with an interest in ITP and can be reached at its e-mail address at aliunehattamam.iai.co.il.

Relevant area(s) of interest: Purpura, Idiopathic Thrombocytopenic, Werlhof Disease

- **ITP People Place**

  Address:

  Telephone: (212) 297-4336 Toll-free: (800) 487-701

  Email: pdsa@pdsa.org

  Web Site: http://www.itppeople.co

  Background: ITP People Place is a web site on the Internet dedicated to providing information, support, resources, and online networking opportunities to individuals with Idiopathic Thrombocytopenia Purpura (ITP). ITP is characterized by abnormally low levels of circulating blood platelets (thrombocytopenia) without a readily apparent cause or underlying disease (idiopathic). The disorder may be characterized by small areas of abnormal bleeding (minor hemorrhages) within skin (dermal) layers or layers below the mucous membranes (submucosal), causing the appearance of small purplish spots on the skin (petechia); bleeding from mucous membranes that may be manifested by nose bleeds, for example; increased susceptibility to bruising; and/or other symptoms. In some cases, affected individuals may exhibit fever, slight enlargement of the spleen (splenomegaly), and/or other characteristics. The ITP People Place site offers understandable information about the potential underlying causes of ITP, symptoms and findings associated with the disorder, current treatments, and research conducted on ITP. The site also provides listings of peer-reviewed medical journal articles in several categories (including ITP in Children, ITP and Pregnancy, ITP in Adults, Gammaglobulin, Splenectomy, Methylprednisone, and Other

Treatments); offers dynamic linkage to other helpful sources of information on the Internet; and offers online visitors the opportunity to participate in several surveys (such as a general ITP survey and a children s survey) whose results are then shared on the site. ITP People Place also offers several online networking opportunities including a Message Board where visitors can read and post messages, questions, and comments and a Mailing List that enables subscribers to receive a listing of others who would like to communicate with one another via e-mail.

Relevant area(s) of interest: Purpura, Idiopathic Thrombocytopenic, Werlhof Disease

- **ITP Society of the Children's Blood Foundation**

  Address: ITP Society of the Children's Blood Foundation Children's Blood Foundation, 333 East 38th Street, New York, NY 10016

  Telephone: (212) 297-4336 Toll-free: (800) 487-701

  Fax: (212) 297-4340

  Background: The ITP Society of the Children's Blood Foundation is a not-for-profit organization dedicated to promoting the welfare of and addressing the issues that affect people with Immune or Idiopathic Thrombocytopenic Purpura (ITP), a condition characterized by deficiency of circulating blood platelets resulting in bleeding into the skin and other organs. The ITP Society was founded in 1994 under the auspices of The Children's Blood Foundation. The Society's goals are to provide patient support and give appropriate referrals; support ongoing medical research to advance the knowledge and treatment of ITP; and educate the public and medical communities about the disorder. The ITP Society provides educational and support materials including fact sheets, brochures, and a booklet entitled 'What's It Called Again?'.

  Relevant area(s) of interest: Purpura, Idiopathic Thrombocytopenic, Werlhof Disease

Finding More Associations

There are a number of directories that list additional medical associations that you may find useful. While not all of these directories will provide different information than what is listed above, by consulting all of them, you will have nearly exhausted all sources for patient associations.

The National Health Information Center (NHIC)

The National Health Information Center (NHIC) offers a free referral service to help people find organizations that provide information about immune thrombocytopenic purpura. For more information, see the NHIC's Web site at **http://www.health.gov/NHIC/** or contact an information specialist by calling 1-800-336-4797.

DIRLINE

A comprehensive source of information on associations is the DIRLINE database maintained by the National Library of Medicine. The database comprises some 10,000 records of organizations, research centers, and government institutes and associations which primarily focus on health and biomedicine. DIRLINE is available via the Internet at the following Web site: **http://dirline.nlm.nih.gov/**. Simply type in "immune thrombocytopenic purpura" (or a synonym) or the name of a topic, and the site will list information contained in the database on all relevant organizations.

The Combined Health Information Database

Another comprehensive source of information on healthcare associations is the Combined Health Information Database. Using the "Detailed Search" option, you will need to limit your search to "Organizations" and "immune thrombocytopenic purpura". Type the following hyperlink into your Web browser: **http://chid.nih.gov/detail/detail.html**. To find associations, use the drop boxes at the bottom of the search page where "You may refine your search by." For publication date, select "All Years." Then, select your preferred language and the format option "Organization Resource Sheet." By making these selections and typing in "immune thrombocytopenic purpura" (or synonyms) into the "For these words:" box, you will only receive results on organizations dealing with immune thrombocytopenic purpura. You should check back periodically with this database since it is updated every 3 months.

The National Organization for Rare Disorders, Inc.

The National Organization for Rare Disorders, Inc. has prepared a Web site that provides, at no charge, lists of associations organized by specific diseases. You can access this database at the following Web site:

http://www.rarediseases.org/cgi-bin/nord/searchpage. Select the option called "Organizational Database (ODB)" and type "immune thrombocytopenic purpura" (or a synonym) in the search box.

Online Support Groups

In addition to support groups, commercial Internet service providers offer forums and chat rooms for people with different illnesses and conditions. WebMD®, for example, offers such a service at their Web site: **http://boards.webmd.com/roundtable**. These online self-help communities can help you connect with a network of people whose concerns are similar to yours. Online support groups are places where people can talk informally. If you read about a novel approach, consult with your doctor or other healthcare providers, as the treatments or discoveries you hear about may not be scientifically proven to be safe and effective. The following Internet links may be of particular interest:

- **Immune thrombocytopenic purpura**
  rarediseases.about.com/cs/itp/

- **The CaF Directory**
  www.cafamily.org.uk/Direct/i12.html

- **Patient UK**
  www.patient.co.uk/selfhelp/blood

Finding Doctors

One of the most important aspects of your treatment will be the relationship between you and your doctor or specialist. All patients with immune thrombocytopenic purpura must go through the process of selecting a physician. While this process will vary from person to person, the Agency for Healthcare Research and Quality makes a number of suggestions, including the following:[12]

- If you are in a managed care plan, check the plan's list of doctors first.

- Ask doctors or other health professionals who work with doctors, such as hospital nurses, for referrals.

---

[12] This section is adapted from the AHRQ: **www.ahrq.gov/consumer/qntascii/qntdr.htm** .

- Call a hospital's doctor referral service, but keep in mind that these services usually refer you to doctors on staff at that particular hospital. The services do not have information on the quality of care that these doctors provide.

- Some local medical societies offer lists of member doctors. Again, these lists do not have information on the quality of care that these doctors provide.

Additional steps you can take to locate doctors include the following:

- Check with the associations listed earlier in this chapter.

- Information on doctors in some states is available on the Internet at **http://www.docboard.org**. This Web site is run by "Administrators in Medicine," a group of state medical board directors.

- The American Board of Medical Specialties can tell you if your doctor is board certified. "Certified" means that the doctor has completed a training program in a specialty and has passed an exam, or "board," to assess his or her knowledge, skills, and experience to provide quality patient care in that specialty. Primary care doctors may also be certified as specialists. The AMBS Web site is located at **http://www.abms.org/newsearch.asp**.[13] You can also contact the ABMS by phone at 1-866-ASK-ABMS.

- You can call the American Medical Association (AMA) at 800-665-2882 for information on training, specialties, and board certification for many licensed doctors in the United States. This information also can be found in "Physician Select" at the AMA's Web site: **http://www.ama-assn.org/aps/amahg.htm**.

If the previous sources did not meet your needs, you may want to log on to the Web site of the National Organization for Rare Disorders (NORD) at **http://www.rarediseases.org/**. NORD maintains a database of doctors with expertise in various rare diseases. The Metabolic Information Network (MIN), 800-945-2188, also maintains a database of physicians with expertise in various metabolic diseases.

---

[13] While board certification is a good measure of a doctor's knowledge, it is possible to receive quality care from doctors who are not board certified.

Selecting Your Doctor[14]

When you have compiled a list of prospective doctors, call each of their offices. First, ask if the doctor accepts your health insurance plan and if he or she is taking new patients. If the doctor is not covered by your plan, ask yourself if you are prepared to pay the extra costs. The next step is to schedule a visit with your chosen physician. During the first visit you will have the opportunity to evaluate your doctor and to find out if you feel comfortable with him or her. Ask yourself, did the doctor:

- Give me a chance to ask questions about immune thrombocytopenic purpura?
- Really listen to my questions?
- Answer in terms I understood?
- Show respect for me?
- Ask me questions?
- Make me feel comfortable?
- Address the health problem(s) I came with?
- Ask me my preferences about different kinds of treatments for immune thrombocytopenic purpura?
- Spend enough time with me?

Trust your instincts when deciding if the doctor is right for you. But remember, it might take time for the relationship to develop. It takes more than one visit for you and your doctor to get to know each other.

Working with Your Doctor[15]

Research has shown that patients who have good relationships with their doctors tend to be more satisfied with their care and have better results. Here are some tips to help you and your doctor become partners:

- You know important things about your symptoms and your health history. Tell your doctor what you think he or she needs to know.

---

[14] This section has been adapted from the AHRQ:
www.ahrq.gov/consumer/qntascii/qntdr.htm.
[15] This section has been adapted from the AHRQ:
www.ahrq.gov/consumer/qntascii/qntdr.htm.

- It is important to tell your doctor personal information, even if it makes you feel embarrassed or uncomfortable.

- Bring a "health history" list with you (and keep it up to date).

- Always bring any medications you are currently taking with you to the appointment, or you can bring a list of your medications including dosage and frequency information. Talk about any allergies or reactions you have had to your medications.

- Tell your doctor about any natural or alternative medicines you are taking.

- Bring other medical information, such as x-ray films, test results, and medical records.

- Ask questions. If you don't, your doctor will assume that you understood everything that was said.

- Write down your questions before your visit. List the most important ones first to make sure that they are addressed.

- Consider bringing a friend with you to the appointment to help you ask questions. This person can also help you understand and/or remember the answers.

- Ask your doctor to draw pictures if you think that this would help you understand.

- Take notes. Some doctors do not mind if you bring a tape recorder to help you remember things, but always ask first.

- Let your doctor know if you need more time. If there is not time that day, perhaps you can speak to a nurse or physician assistant on staff or schedule a telephone appointment.

- Take information home. Ask for written instructions. Your doctor may also have brochures and audio and videotapes that can help you.

- After leaving the doctor's office, take responsibility for your care. If you have questions, call. If your symptoms get worse or if you have problems with your medication, call. If you had tests and do not hear from your doctor, call for your test results. If your doctor recommended that you have certain tests, schedule an appointment to get them done. If your doctor said you should see an additional specialist, make an appointment.

By following these steps, you will enhance the relationship you will have with your physician.

Broader Health-Related Resources

In addition to the references above, the NIH has set up guidance Web sites that can help patients find healthcare professionals. These include:[16]

- Caregivers:
  http://www.nlm.nih.gov/medlineplus/caregivers.html

- Choosing a Doctor or Healthcare Service:
  http://www.nlm.nih.gov/medlineplus/choosingadoctororhealthcareserv ice.html

- Hospitals and Health Facilities:
  http://www.nlm.nih.gov/medlineplus/healthfacilities.html

Vocabulary Builder

The following vocabulary builder provides definitions of words used in this chapter that have not been defined in previous chapters:

Anemia: A reduction in the number of circulating erythrocytes or in the quantity of hemoglobin. [NIH]

Hemorrhage: Bleeding or escape of blood from a vessel. [NIH]

Splenomegaly: Enlargement of the spleen. [EU]

Thalassemia: A group of hereditary hemolytic anemias in which there is decreased synthesis of one or more hemoglobin polypeptide chains. There are several genetic types with clinical pictures ranging from barely detectable hematologic abnormality to severe and fatal anemia. [NIH]

---

[16] You can access this information at:
http://www.nlm.nih.gov/medlineplus/healthsystem.html.

CHAPTER 3. CLINICAL TRIALS AND IMMUNE THROMBOCYTOPENIC PURPURA

Overview

Very few medical conditions have a single treatment. The basic treatment guidelines that your physician has discussed with you, or those that you have found using the techniques discussed in Chapter 1, may provide you with all that you will require. For some patients, current treatments can be enhanced with new or innovative techniques currently under investigation. In this chapter, we will describe how clinical trials work and show you how to keep informed of trials concerning immune thrombocytopenic purpura.

What Is a Clinical Trial? [17]

Clinical trials involve the participation of people in medical research. Most medical research begins with studies in test tubes and on animals. Treatments that show promise in these early studies may then be tried with people. The only sure way to find out whether a new treatment is safe, effective, and better than other treatments for immune thrombocytopenic purpura is to try it on patients in a clinical trial.

---

[17] The discussion in this chapter has been adapted from the NIH and the NEI: **www.nei.nih.gov/netrials/ctivr.htm**.

What Kinds of Clinical Trials Are There?

Clinical trials are carried out in three phases:

- **Phase I.** Researchers first conduct Phase I trials with small numbers of patients and healthy volunteers. If the new treatment is a medication, researchers also try to determine how much of it can be given safely.

- **Phase II.** Researchers conduct Phase II trials in small numbers of patients to find out the effect of a new treatment on immune thrombocytopenic purpura.

- **Phase III.** Finally, researchers conduct Phase III trials to find out how new treatments for immune thrombocytopenic purpura compare with standard treatments already being used. Phase III trials also help to determine if new treatments have any side effects. These trials--which may involve hundreds, perhaps thousands, of people--can also compare new treatments with no treatment.

How Is a Clinical Trial Conducted?

Various organizations support clinical trials at medical centers, hospitals, universities, and doctors' offices across the United States. The "principal investigator" is the researcher in charge of the study at each facility participating in the clinical trial. Most clinical trial researchers are medical doctors, academic researchers, and specialists. The "clinic coordinator" knows all about how the study works and makes all the arrangements for your visits.

All doctors and researchers who take part in the study on immune thrombocytopenic purpura carefully follow a detailed treatment plan called a protocol. This plan fully explains how the doctors will treat you in the study. The "protocol" ensures that all patients are treated in the same way, no matter where they receive care.

Clinical trials are controlled. This means that researchers compare the effects of the new treatment with those of the standard treatment. In some cases, when no standard treatment exists, the new treatment is compared with no treatment. Patients who receive the new treatment are in the treatment group. Patients who receive a standard treatment or no treatment are in the "control" group. In some clinical trials, patients in the treatment group get a new medication while those in the control group get a placebo. A placebo is a harmless substance, a "dummy" pill, that has no effect on immune thrombocytopenic purpura. In other clinical trials, where a new surgery or device (not a medicine) is being tested, patients in the control group may receive a "sham treatment." This treatment, like a placebo, has no effect on immune thrombocytopenic purpura and does not harm patients.

Researchers assign patients "randomly" to the treatment or control group. This is like flipping a coin to decide which patients are in each group. If you choose to participate in a clinical trial, you will not know which group you will be appointed to. The chance of any patient getting the new treatment is about 50 percent. You cannot request to receive the new treatment instead of the placebo or sham treatment. Often, you will not know until the study is over whether you have been in the treatment group or the control group. This is called a "masked" study. In some trials, neither doctors nor patients know who is getting which treatment. This is called a "double masked" study. These types of trials help to ensure that the perceptions of the patients or doctors will not affect the study results.

Natural History Studies

Unlike clinical trials in which patient volunteers may receive new treatments, natural history studies provide important information to researchers on how immune thrombocytopenic purpura develops over time. A natural history study follows patient volunteers to see how factors such as age, sex, race, or family history might make some people more or less at risk for immune thrombocytopenic purpura. A natural history study may also tell researchers if diet, lifestyle, or occupation affects how a disease or disorder develops and progresses. Results from these studies provide information that helps answer questions such as: How fast will a disease or disorder usually progress? How bad will the condition become? Will treatment be needed?

What Is Expected of Patients in a Clinical Trial?

Not everyone can take part in a clinical trial for a specific disease or disorder. Each study enrolls patients with certain features or eligibility criteria. These criteria may include the type and stage of disease or disorder, as well as, the age and previous treatment history of the patient. You or your doctor can contact the sponsoring organization to find out more about specific clinical trials and their eligibility criteria. If you are interested in joining a clinical trial, your doctor must contact one of the trial's investigators and provide details about your diagnosis and medical history.

If you participate in a clinical trial, you may be required to have a number of medical tests. You may also need to take medications and/or undergo surgery. Depending upon the treatment and the examination procedure, you may be required to receive inpatient hospital care. Or, you may have to return to the medical facility for follow-up examinations. These exams help find out how well the treatment is working. Follow-up studies can take months or years. However, the success of the clinical trial often depends on learning what happens to patients over a long period of time. Only patients who continue to return for follow-up examinations can provide this important long-term information.

Recent Trials on Immune Thrombocytopenic Purpura

The National Institutes of Health and other organizations sponsor trials on various diseases and disorders. Because funding for research goes to the medical areas that show promising research opportunities, it is not possible for the NIH or others to sponsor clinical trials for every disease and disorder at all times. The following lists recent trials dedicated to immune thrombocytopenic purpura.[18] If the trial listed by the NIH is still recruiting, you may be eligible. If it is no longer recruiting or has been completed, then you can contact the sponsors to learn more about the study and, if published, the results. Further information on the trial is available at the Web site indicated. Please note that some trials may no longer be recruiting patients or are otherwise closed. Before contacting sponsors of a clinical trial, consult with your physician who can help you determine if you might benefit from participation.

- **Autologous Peripheral Blood Stem Cell Transplantation in Patients With Life Threatening Autoimmune Diseases**

    Condition(s): Purpura, Schoenlein-Henoch; Graft Versus Host Disease; Anemia, Hemolytic, Autoimmune; Rheumatoid Arthritis; Churg-Strauss Syndrome; Hypersensitivity Vasculitis; Wegener's Granulomatosis; Systemic Lupus Erythematosus; Giant Cell Arteritis; Pure Red Cell Aplasia; Juvenile Rheumatoid Arthritis; Polyarteritis Nodosa; Autoimmune Thrombocytopenic Purpura; Takayasu Arteritis

    Study Status: This study is currently recruiting patients.

    Sponsor(s): Fairview University Medical Center

    Purpose - Excerpt: Objectives: I. Determine whether there is prompt engraftment after autologous peripheral blood stem cell transplantation using filgrastim (G-CSF) mobilization in patients with life threatening

---

[18] These are listed at www.ClinicalTrials.gov.

autoimmune diseases. II. Determine the kinetics of T- and B-cell immune reconstitution after a combination of timed plasmapheresis, high dose cyclophosphamide and total lymphoid irradiation, and posttransplant immunosuppression with cyclosporine in these patients. III. Determine whether this treatment regimen beneficially influences the clinical course of these patients.

Study Type: Interventional

Contact(s): Minnesota; Fairview University Medical Center, Minneapolis, Minnesota, 55455, United States; Recruiting; Arne Slungaard 612-273-2800. Study chairs or principal investigators: Arne Slungaard, Study Chair; Fairview University Medical Center

Web Site: http://clinicaltrials.gov/ct/gui/c/w1b/show/NCT00006055

- **A Phase I Study of Recombinant Human CD4 Immunoglobulin G (rCD4-lgG) in Patients with HIV-Associated Immune Thrombocytopenic Purpura**

Condition(s): Immune thrombocytopenic purpura (ITP); HIV Infections

Study Status: This study is no longer recruiting patients.

Sponsor(s): Genentech

Purpose - Excerpt: To test the effectiveness of recombinant human CD4 Immunoglobulin G (CD4-IgG) in the treatment of HIV-associated immune thrombocytopenic purpura in patients with all levels of HIV infection.

Phase(s): Phase I

Study Type: Interventional

Contact(s): California; San Francisco Gen Hosp, San Francisco, California, 941102859, United States

Web Site: http://clinicaltrials.gov/ct/gui/c/w1b/show/NCT00002250

- **Phase II Study of Rituximab in Patients With Immune Thrombocytopenic Purpura**

Condition(s): Purpura, Thrombocytopenic, Idiopathic

Study Status: This study is no longer recruiting patients.

Sponsor(s): UAB Comprehensive Cancer Center

Purpose - Excerpt: Objectives: I. Determine the response rate and response duration to rituximab in patients with immune thrombocytopenic purpura. II. Evaluate the toxicity associated with this treatment regimen in these patients. III. Evaluate the alteration in antiplatelet antibody with this treatment regimen in these patients.

Phase(s): Phase II

Study Type: Interventional

Contact(s): Alabama; University of Alabama Comprehensive Cancer Center, Birmingham, Alabama, 35294, United States; Mansoor Noorali Saleh 205-975-9025. Study chairs or principal investigators: Mansoor Noorali Saleh, Study Chair; UAB Comprehensive Cancer Center

Web Site: http://clinicaltrials.gov/ct/gui/c/w1b/show/NCT00005652

Benefits and Risks[19]

What Are the Benefits of Participating in a Clinical Trial?

If you are interested in a clinical trial, it is important to realize that your participation can bring many benefits to you and society at large:

- A new treatment could be more effective than the current treatment for immune thrombocytopenic purpura. Although only half of the participants in a clinical trial receive the experimental treatment, if the new treatment is proved to be more effective and safer than the current treatment, then those patients who did not receive the new treatment during the clinical trial may be among the first to benefit from it when the study is over.

- If the treatment is effective, then it may improve health or prevent diseases or disorders.

- Clinical trial patients receive the highest quality of medical care. Experts watch them closely during the study and may continue to follow them after the study is over.

- People who take part in trials contribute to scientific discoveries that may help other people with immune thrombocytopenic purpura. In cases where certain diseases or disorders run in families, your participation may lead to better care or prevention for your family members.

---

[19] This section has been adapted from ClinicalTrials.gov, a service of the National Institutes of Health:
http://www.clinicaltrials.gov/ct/gui/c/a1r/info/whatis?JServSessionIdzone_ct=9jmun6f2
91.

The Informed Consent

Once you agree to take part in a clinical trial, you will be asked to sign an "informed consent." This document explains a clinical trial's risks and benefits, the researcher's expectations of you, and your rights as a patient.

What Are the Risks?

Clinical trials may involve risks as well as benefits. Whether or not a new treatment will work cannot be known ahead of time. There is always a chance that a new treatment may not work better than a standard treatment. There is also the possibility that it may be harmful. The treatment you receive may cause side effects that are serious enough to require medical attention.

How Is Patient Safety Protected?

Clinical trials can raise fears of the unknown. Understanding the safeguards that protect patients can ease some of these fears. Before a clinical trial begins, researchers must get approval from their hospital's Institutional Review Board (IRB), an advisory group that makes sure a clinical trial is designed to protect patient safety. During a clinical trial, doctors will closely watch you to see if the treatment is working and if you are experiencing any side effects. All the results are carefully recorded and reviewed. In many cases, experts from the Data and Safety Monitoring Committee carefully monitor each clinical trial and can recommend that a study be stopped at any time. You will only be asked to take part in a clinical trial as a volunteer giving informed consent.

What Are a Patient's Rights in a Clinical Trial?

If you are eligible for a clinical trial, you will be given information to help you decide whether or not you want to participate. As a patient, you have the right to:

• Information on all known risks and benefits of the treatments in the study.

• Know how the researchers plan to carry out the study, for how long, and where.

• Know what is expected of you.

- Know any costs involved for you or your insurance provider.

- Know before any of your medical or personal information is shared with other researchers involved in the clinical trial.

- Talk openly with doctors and ask any questions.

After you join a clinical trial, you have the right to:

- Leave the study at any time. Participation is strictly voluntary. However, you should not enroll if you do not plan to complete the study.

- Receive any new information about the new treatment.

- Continue to ask questions and get answers.

- Maintain your privacy. Your name will not appear in any reports based on the study.

- Know whether you participated in the treatment group or the control group (once the study has been completed).

What about Costs?

In some clinical trials, the research facility pays for treatment costs and other associated expenses. You or your insurance provider may have to pay for costs that are considered standard care. These things may include inpatient hospital care, laboratory and other tests, and medical procedures. You also may need to pay for travel between your home and the clinic. You should find out about costs before committing to participation in the trial. If you have health insurance, find out exactly what it will cover. If you don't have health insurance, or if your insurance company will not cover your costs, talk to the clinic staff about other options for covering the cost of your care.

What Should You Ask before Deciding to Join a Clinical Trial?

Questions you should ask when thinking about joining a clinical trial include the following:

- What is the purpose of the clinical trial?

- What are the standard treatments for immune thrombocytopenic purpura? Why do researchers think the new treatment may be better? What is likely to happen to me with or without the new treatment?

- What tests and treatments will I need? Will I need surgery? Medication? Hospitalization?

- How long will the treatment last? How often will I have to come back for follow-up exams?

- What are the treatment's possible benefits to my condition? What are the short- and long-term risks? What are the possible side effects?

- Will the treatment be uncomfortable? Will it make me feel sick? If so, for how long?

- How will my health be monitored?

- Where will I need to go for the clinical trial? How will I get there?

- How much will it cost to be in the study? What costs are covered by the study? How much will my health insurance cover?

- Will I be able to see my own doctor? Who will be in charge of my care?

- Will taking part in the study affect my daily life? Do I have time to participate?

- How do I feel about taking part in a clinical trial? Are there family members or friends who may benefit from my contributions to new medical knowledge?

Keeping Current on Clinical Trials

Various government agencies maintain databases on trials. The U.S. National Institutes of Health, through the National Library of Medicine, has developed ClinicalTrials.gov to provide patients, family members, and physicians with current information about clinical research across the broadest number of diseases and conditions.

The site was launched in February 2000 and currently contains approximately 5,700 clinical studies in over 59,000 locations worldwide, with most studies being conducted in the United States. ClinicalTrials.gov receives about 2 million hits per month and hosts approximately 5,400 visitors daily. To access this database, simply go to their Web site (**www.clinicaltrials.gov**) and search by "immune thrombocytopenic purpura" (or synonyms).

While ClinicalTrials.gov is the most comprehensive listing of NIH-supported clinical trials available, not all trials are in the database. The database is updated regularly, so clinical trials are continually being added. The following is a list of specialty databases affiliated with the National Institutes of Health that offer additional information on trials:

- For clinical studies at the Warren Grant Magnuson Clinical Center located in Bethesda, Maryland, visit their Web site: **http://clinicalstudies.info.nih.gov/**

- For clinical studies conducted at the Bayview Campus in Baltimore, Maryland, visit their Web site: **http://www.jhbmc.jhu.edu/studies/index.html**

- For heart, lung and blood trials, visit the Web page of the National Heart, Lung and Blood Institute: **http://www.nhlbi.nih.gov/studies/index.htm**

General References

The following references describe clinical trials and experimental medical research. They have been selected to ensure that they are likely to be available from your local or online bookseller or university medical library. These references are usually written for healthcare professionals, so you may consider consulting with a librarian or bookseller who might recommend a particular reference. The following includes some of the most readily available references (sorted alphabetically by title; hyperlinks provide rankings, information and reviews at Amazon.com):

- **A Guide to Patient Recruitment : Today's Best Practices & Proven Strategies** by Diana L. Anderson; Paperback - 350 pages (2001), CenterWatch, Inc.; ISBN: 1930624115; **http://www.amazon.com/exec/obidos/ASIN/1930624115/icongroupinterna**

- **A Step-By-Step Guide to Clinical Trials** by Marilyn Mulay, R.N., M.S., OCN; Spiral-bound - 143 pages Spiral edition (2001), Jones & Bartlett Pub; ISBN: 0763715697; **http://www.amazon.com/exec/obidos/ASIN/0763715697/icongroupinterna**

- **The CenterWatch Directory of Drugs in Clinical Trials** by CenterWatch; Paperback - 656 pages (2000), CenterWatch, Inc.; ISBN: 0967302935; **http://www.amazon.com/exec/obidos/ASIN/0967302935/icongroupinterna**

- **The Complete Guide to Informed Consent in Clinical Trials** by Terry Hartnett (Editor); Paperback - 164 pages (2000), PharmSource Information Services, Inc.; ISBN: 0970153309; **http://www.amazon.com/exec/obidos/ASIN/0970153309/icongroupinterna**

- **Dictionary for Clinical Trials** by Simon Day; Paperback - 228 pages (1999), John Wiley & Sons; ISBN: 0471985961; **http://www.amazon.com/exec/obidos/ASIN/0471985961/icongroupinterna**

- **Extending Medicare Reimbursement in Clinical Trials** by Institute of Medicine Staff (Editor), et al; Paperback 1st edition (2000), National Academy Press; ISBN: 0309068886; http://www.amazon.com/exec/obidos/ASIN/0309068886/icongroupinterna

- **Handbook of Clinical Trials** by Marcus Flather (Editor); Paperback (2001), Remedica Pub Ltd; ISBN: 1901346293; http://www.amazon.com/exec/obidos/ASIN/1901346293/icongroupinterna

Vocabulary Builder

The following vocabulary builder gives definitions of words used in this chapter that have not been defined in previous chapters:

Aplasia: Lack of development of an organ or tissue, or of the cellular products from an organ or tissue. [EU]

Arteritis: Inflammation of an artery. [NIH]

Hypersensitivity: A state of altered reactivity in which the body reacts with an exaggerated immune response to a foreign substance. Hypersensitivity reactions are classified as immediate or delayed, types I and IV, respectively, in the Gell and Coombs classification (q.v.) of immune responses. [EU]

Kinetic: Pertaining to or producing motion. [EU]

Mobilization: The process of making a fixed part or stored substance mobile, as by separating a part from surrounding structures to make it accessible for an operative procedure or by causing release into the circulation for body use of a substance stored in the body. [EU]

Plasmapheresis: Procedure whereby plasma is separated and extracted from anticoagulated whole blood and the red cells retransfused to the donor. Plasmapheresis is also employed for therapeutic use. [NIH]

Recombinant: 1. a cell or an individual with a new combination of genes not found together in either parent; usually applied to linked genes. [EU]

Reconstitution: 1. a type of regeneration in which a new organ forms by the rearrangement of tissues rather than from new formation at an injured surface. 2. the restoration to original form of a substance previously altered for preservation and storage, as the restoration to a liquid state of blood serum or plasma that has been dried and stored. [EU]

Rheumatoid: Resembling rheumatism. [EU]

Toxicity: The quality of being poisonous, especially the degree of virulence of a toxic microbe or of a poison. [EU]

Vasculitis: Inflammation of a vessel, angiitis. [EU]

PART II: ADDITIONAL RESOURCES AND ADVANCED MATERIAL

ABOUT PART II

In Part II, we introduce you to additional resources and advanced research on immune thrombocytopenic purpura. All too often, patients who conduct their own research are overwhelmed by the difficulty in finding and organizing information. The purpose of the following chapters is to provide you an organized and structured format to help you find additional information resources on immune thrombocytopenic purpura. In Part II, as in Part I, our objective is not to interpret the latest advances on immune thrombocytopenic purpura or render an opinion. Rather, our goal is to give you access to original research and to increase your awareness of sources you may not have already considered. In this way, you will come across the advanced materials often referred to in pamphlets, books, or other general works. Once again, some of this material is technical in nature, so consultation with a professional familiar with immune thrombocytopenic purpura is suggested.

CHAPTER 4. STUDIES ON IMMUNE THROMBOCYTOPENIC PURPURA

Overview

Every year, academic studies are published on immune thrombocytopenic purpura or related conditions. Broadly speaking, there are two types of studies. The first are peer reviewed. Generally, the content of these studies has been reviewed by scientists or physicians. Peer-reviewed studies are typically published in scientific journals and are usually available at medical libraries. The second type of studies is non-peer reviewed. These works include summary articles that do not use or report scientific results. These often appear in the popular press, newsletters, or similar periodicals.

In this chapter, we will show you how to locate peer-reviewed references and studies on immune thrombocytopenic purpura. We will begin by discussing research that has been summarized and is free to view by the public via the Internet. We then show you how to generate a bibliography on immune thrombocytopenic purpura and teach you how to keep current on new studies as they are published or undertaken by the scientific community.

Federally-Funded Research on Immune Thrombocytopenic Purpura

The U.S. Government supports a variety of research studies relating to immune thrombocytopenic purpura and associated conditions. These studies are tracked by the Office of Extramural Research at the National

Institutes of Health.[20] CRISP (Computerized Retrieval of Information on Scientific Projects) is a searchable database of federally-funded biomedical research projects conducted at universities, hospitals, and other institutions. Visit the site at **http://commons.cit.nih.gov/crisp3/CRISP.Generate_Ticket**. You can perform targeted searches by various criteria including geography, date, as well as topics related to immune thrombocytopenic purpura and related conditions

For most of the studies, the agencies reporting into CRISP provide summaries or abstracts. As opposed to clinical trial research using patients, many federally-funded studies use animals or simulated models to explore immune thrombocytopenic purpura and related conditions. In some cases, therefore, it may be difficult to understand how some basic or fundamental research could eventually translate into medical practice. The following sample is typical of the type of information found when searching the CRISP database for immune thrombocytopenic purpura:

- **Project Title: Autologous Platelets In Immune Thrombocytopenic Purpura**

  Principal Investigator & Institution: Bell, William; ; Johns Hopkins University 3400 N Charles St Baltimore, Md 21218

  Timing: Fiscal Year 2000; Project Start 1-OCT-1975; Project End 0-NOV-2004

  Summary: The primary aim of this study to show that oral tolerance can be used to treat ITP. Orally introduced platelets can increase the platelet count of ITP patients.

  Website: http://commons.cit.nih.gov/crisp3/CRISP.Generate_Ticket

- **Project Title: Rituxan In Treatment Of Immune Thrombocytopenic Purpura**

  Principal Investigator & Institution: Lobuglio, Albert F.; Professor/Director; University of Alabama at Birmingham Uab Station Birmingham, Al 35294

  Timing: Fiscal Year 2000; Project Start 1-DEC-1978; Project End 0-NOV-2002

  Summary: We have to date treated 11 patients with clinical ITP. 7 patients with prior splenectomy and 4 who have not been

---

[20] Healthcare projects are funded by the National Institutes of Health (NIH), Substance Abuse and Mental Health Services (SAMHSA), Health Resources and Services Administration (HRSA), Food and Drug Administration (FDA), Centers for Disease Control and Prevention (CDCP), Agency for Healthcare Research and Quality (AHRQ), and Office of Assistant Secretary of Health (OASH).

splenectomized. 3 of 11 responded to Rituxan therapy and the study is ongoing to accrue a total of 20 patients.

Website: http://commons.cit.nih.gov/crisp3/CRISP.Generate_Ticket

- **Project Title: Autoimmune Hemolytic Anemia And Expression Of Ig Genes**

Principal Investigator & Institution: Kipps, Thomas J.; Professor and Head, Division of Hematolo; University of California San Diego Gilman & La Jolla Village Dr San Diego, Ca 92093

Timing: Fiscal Year 2000; Project Start 1-MAR-1974; Project End 0-NOV-2004

Summary: Identify the IgVH genes expressed by leukemia cells of patients with chronic lymphocytic leukemia and then evaluate such patients for the development of autoimmune hemolytic anemia or immune thrombocytopenic purpura.

Website: http://commons.cit.nih.gov/crisp3/CRISP.Generate_Ticket

- **Project Title: IGIV-Chromatography In PTS w/Idiopathic Thrombocytopenic Purpura**

Principal Investigator & Institution: Cooper, Herbert A.; ; University of North Carolina Chapel Hill Chapel Hill, Nc 27514

Timing: Fiscal Year 2000; Project Start 1-OCT-1974; Project End 0-NOV-2002

Summary: The purpose of this research study is to determine the safety and outcome of treatment with an investigational immune globulin product: Immune Globulin Intravenous (Human) manufactured using chromatography as part of the purification process (IGIV-C, 10%) in patients with confirmed Idiopathic (Immune) Thrombocytopenic Purpura (ITP). This condition results in low platelet counts because of increased destruction of platelets (blood cells important for blood clotting) by the body's immune system. Intravenous immune globulin is given to patients with immune thrombocytopenic purpura (ITP) when it is important to raise the level of platelets circulating in the blood stream. Intravenous immune globulin was first licensed for medical use in the United States in 1981, and immune globulin products in various concentrations and from different preparation/purification methods have been licensed for use in the treatment of ITP since then. In this study, Bayer Corporation is evaluating an intravenous immune globulin preparation that is manufactured in a new way. The product is purer than Bayer's prevous preparations of IGIV and more closely reflects the types of immunoglobulin found in normal blood. The manufacturing process also includes a new viral inactivation step that uses a technique called chromatography. The new product will be referred to a IGIV-C, 10%. Although older formulations of Bayer's intravenous immune globulin have been approved for use by the Federal Drug Administration, the new product to be used in this study is not yet approved. Information learned in this study will become part of an application to license this product (IGIV-C, 10%) in the United States and around the world.

Website: http://commons.cit.nih.gov/crisp3/CRISP.Generate_Ticket

E-Journals: PubMed Central[21]

PubMed Central (PMC) is a digital archive of life sciences journal literature developed and managed by the National Center for Biotechnology Information (NCBI) at the U.S. National Library of Medicine (NLM).[22] Access to this growing archive of e-journals is free and unrestricted.[23] To search, go to **http://www.pubmedcentral.nih.gov/index.html#search**, and type "immune thrombocytopenic purpura" (or synonyms) into the search box. This search gives you access to full-text articles. The following is a sample of items found for immune thrombocytopenic purpura in the PubMed Central database:

- **Sequestration of Anti-Platelet GPIIIa Antibody in Rheumatoid Factor Immune Complexes of Human Immunodeficiency Virus 1 Thrombocytopenic Patients** by S Karatkin, MA Nardi, and KB Hymes; 1995 March 14
  http://www.pubmedcentral.nih.gov/articlerender.fcgi?rendertype=abstract&artid=42464

The National Library of Medicine: PubMed

One of the quickest and most comprehensive ways to find academic studies in both English and other languages is to use PubMed, maintained by the

---

[21] Adapted from the National Library of Medicine:
http://www.pubmedcentral.nih.gov/about/intro.html.
[22] With PubMed Central, NCBI is taking the lead in preservation and maintenance of open access to electronic literature, just as NLM has done for decades with printed biomedical literature. PubMed Central aims to become a world-class library of the digital age.
[23] The value of PubMed Central, in addition to its role as an archive, lies the availability of data from diverse sources stored in a common format in a single repository. Many journals already have online publishing operations, and there is a growing tendency to publish material online only, to the exclusion of print.

National Library of Medicine. The advantage of PubMed over previously mentioned sources is that it covers a greater number of domestic and foreign references. It is also free to the public.[24] If the publisher has a Web site that offers full text of its journals, PubMed will provide links to that site, as well as to sites offering other related data. User registration, a subscription fee, or some other type of fee may be required to access the full text of articles in some journals.

To generate your own bibliography of studies dealing with immune thrombocytopenic purpura, simply go to the PubMed Web site at **www.ncbi.nlm.nih.gov/pubmed**. Type "immune thrombocytopenic purpura" (or synonyms) into the search box, and click "Go." The following is the type of output you can expect from PubMed for "immune thrombocytopenic purpura" (hyperlinks lead to article summaries):

- **Immunosuppressive therapy of idiopathic thrombocytopenic purpura.**
  Author(s): Caplan SN, Berkman EM.
  Source: The Medical Clinics of North America. 1976 September; 60(5): 971-86. Review.
  http://www.ncbi.nlm.nih.gov:80/entrez/query.fcgi?cmd=Retrieve&db=PubMed&list_uids=781417&dopt=Abstract

- **Overview of idiopathic thrombocytopenic purpura: new approach to refractory patients.**
  Author(s): Bussel JB.
  Source: Seminars in Oncology. 2000 December; 27(6 Suppl 12): 91-8. Review.
  http://www.ncbi.nlm.nih.gov:80/entrez/query.fcgi?cmd=Retrieve&db=PubMed&list_uids=11226007&dopt=Abstract

Vocabulary Builder

Adjuvant: A substance which aids another, such as an auxiliary remedy; in immunology, nonspecific stimulator (e.g., BCG vaccine) of the immune response. [EU]

Agonist: In anatomy, a prime mover. In pharmacology, a drug that has

---

[24] PubMed was developed by the National Center for Biotechnology Information (NCBI) at the National Library of Medicine (NLM) at the National Institutes of Health (NIH). The PubMed database was developed in conjunction with publishers of biomedical literature as a search tool for accessing literature citations and linking to full-text journal articles at Web sites of participating publishers. Publishers that participate in PubMed supply NLM with their citations electronically prior to or at the time of publication.

affinity for and stimulates physiologic activity at cell receptors normally stimulated by naturally occurring substances. [EU]

Anatomical: Pertaining to anatomy, or to the structure of the organism. [EU]

Anergy: Absence of immune response to particular substances. [NIH]

Antibiotic: A drug that kills or inhibits the growth of bacteria. [NIH]

Antigen: Any substance which is capable, under appropriate conditions, of inducing a specific immune response and of reacting with the products of that response, that is, with specific antibody or specifically sensitized T-lymphocytes, or both. Antigens may be soluble substances, such as toxins and foreign proteins, or particulate, such as bacteria and tissue cells; however, only the portion of the protein or polysaccharide molecule known as the antigenic determinant (q.v.) combines with antibody or a specific receptor on a lymphocyte. Abbreviated Ag. [EU]

Arrestin: A 48-Kd protein of the outer segment of the retinal rods and a component of the phototransduction cascade. Arrestin quenches G-protein activation by binding to phosphorylated photolyzed rhodopsin. Arrestin causes experimental autoimmune uveitis when injected into laboratory animals. [NIH]

Assay: Determination of the amount of a particular constituent of a mixture, or of the biological or pharmacological potency of a drug. [EU]

Atopic: Pertaining to an atopen or to atopy; allergic. [EU]

Autoimmunity: Process whereby the immune system reacts against the body's own tissues. Autoimmunity may produce or be caused by autoimmune diseases. [NIH]

Candidiasis: Infection with a fungus of the genus Candida. It is usually a superficial infection of the moist cutaneous areas of the body, and is generally caused by C. albicans; it most commonly involves the skin (dermatocandidiasis), oral mucous membranes (thrush, def. 1), respiratory tract (bronchocandidiasis), and vagina (vaginitis). Rarely there is a systemic infection or endocarditis. Called also moniliasis, candidosis, oidiomycosis, and formerly blastodendriosis. [EU]

Cardiac: Pertaining to the heart. [EU]

Cervical: Pertaining to the neck, or to the neck of any organ or structure. [EU]

Chemotherapy: The treatment of disease by means of chemicals that have a specific toxic effect upon the disease - producing microorganisms or that selectively destroy cancerous tissue. [EU]

Cocaine: An alkaloid ester extracted from the leaves of plants including coca. It is a local anesthetic and vasoconstrictor and is clinically used for that purpose, particularly in the eye, ear, nose, and throat. It also has powerful central nervous system effects similar to the amphetamines and is a drug of abuse. Cocaine, like amphetamines, acts by multiple mechanisms on brain catecholaminergic neurons; the mechanism of its reinforcing effects is thought to involve inhibition of dopamine uptake. [NIH]

Concomitant: Accompanying; accessory; joined with another. [EU]

Cytokines: Non-antibody proteins secreted by inflammatory leukocytes and some non-leukocytic cells, that act as intercellular mediators. They differ from classical hormones in that they are produced by a number of tissue or cell types rather than by specialized glands. They generally act locally in a paracrine or autocrine rather than endocrine manner. [NIH]

Degenerative: Undergoing degeneration : tending to degenerate; having the character of or involving degeneration; causing or tending to cause degeneration. [EU]

Dementia: An acquired organic mental disorder with loss of intellectual abilities of sufficient severity to interfere with social or occupational functioning. The dysfunction is multifaceted and involves memory, behavior, personality, judgment, attention, spatial relations, language, abstract thought, and other executive functions. The intellectual decline is usually progressive, and initially spares the level of consciousness. [NIH]

Dendritic: 1. branched like a tree. 2. pertaining to or possessing dendrites. [EU]

Dermatitis: Inflammation of the skin. [EU]

Efficacy: The extent to which a specific intervention, procedure, regimen, or service produces a beneficial result under ideal conditions. Ideally, the determination of efficacy is based on the results of a randomized control trial. [NIH]

Endothelium: The layer of epithelial cells that lines the cavities of the heart and of the blood and lymph vessels, and the serous cavities of the body, originating from the mesoderm. [EU]

Endotoxin: Toxin from cell walls of bacteria. [NIH]

Epithelium: The covering of internal and external surfaces of the body, including the lining of vessels and other small cavities. It consists of cells joined by small amounts of cementing substances. Epithelium is classified into types on the basis of the number of layers deep and the shape of the superficial cells. [EU]

Epitopes: Sites on an antigen that interact with specific antibodies. [NIH]

Etoposide: A semisynthetic derivative of podophyllotoxin that exhibits antitumor activity. Etoposide inhibits DNA synthesis by forming a complex with topoisomerase II and DNA. This complex induces breaks in double stranded DNA and prevents repair by topoisomerase II binding.

Accumulated breaks in DNA prevent entry into the mitotic phase of cell division, and lead to cell death. Etoposide acts primarily in the G2 and S phases of the cell cycle. [NIH]

Glomerular: Pertaining to or of the nature of a glomerulus, especially a renal glomerulus. [EU]

Glomerulonephritis: A variety of nephritis characterized by inflammation of the capillary loops in the glomeruli of the kidney. It occurs in acute, subacute, and chronic forms and may be secondary to haemolytic streptococcal infection. Evidence also supports possible immune or autoimmune mechanisms. [EU]

Haemostasis: The arrest of bleeding, either by the physiological properties of vasoconstriction and coagulation or by surgical means. [EU]

Herpes: Any inflammatory skin disease caused by a herpesvirus and characterized by the formation of clusters of small vesicles. When used alone, the term may refer to herpes simplex or to herpes zoster. [EU]

Homeostasis: A tendency to stability in the normal body states (internal environment) of the organism. It is achieved by a system of control mechanisms activated by negative feedback; e.g. a high level of carbon dioxide in extracellular fluid triggers increased pulmonary ventilation, which in turn causes a decrease in carbon dioxide concentration. [EU]

Humoral: Of, relating to, proceeding from, or involving a bodily humour - now often used of endocrine factors as opposed to neural or somatic. [EU]

Immunity: The condition of being immune; the protection against infectious disease conferred either by the immune response generated by immunization or previous infection or by other nonimmunologic factors (innate i.). [EU]

Immunization: Protection from disease by administering vaccines that induce the body to form antibodies against infectious agents. [NIH]

Induction: The act or process of inducing or causing to occur, especially the production of a specific morphogenetic effect in the developing embryo through the influence of evocators or organizers, or the production of anaesthesia or unconsciousness by use of appropriate agents. [EU]

Inflammation: Response of the body tissues to injury; typical signs are swelling, redness, and pain. [NIH]

Influenza: An acute viral infection involving the respiratory tract. It is marked by inflammation of the nasal mucosa, the pharynx, and conjunctiva, and by headache and severe, often generalized, myalgia. [NIH]

Lesion: Any pathological or traumatic discontinuity of tissue or loss of function of a part. [EU]

Listeria: A genus of bacteria which may be found in the feces of animals and man, on vegetation, and in silage. Its species are parasitic on cold-blooded and warm-blooded animals, including man. [NIH]

Localization: 1. the determination of the site or place of any process or lesion. 2. restriction to a circumscribed or limited area. 3. prelocalization. [EU]

Mediate: Indirect; accomplished by the aid of an intervening medium. [EU]

Mediator: An object or substance by which something is mediated, such as (1) a structure of the nervous system that transmits impulses eliciting a specific response; (2) a chemical substance (transmitter substance) that induces activity in an excitable tissue, such as nerve or muscle; or (3) a substance released from cells as the result of the interaction of antigen with antibody or by the action of antigen with a sensitized lymphocyte. [EU]

Microbiology: The study of microorganisms such as fungi, bacteria, algae, archaea, and viruses. [NIH]

Microscopy: The application of microscope magnification to the study of materials that cannot be properly seen by the unaided eye. [NIH]

Molecular: Of, pertaining to, or composed of molecules : a very small mass of matter. [EU]

Morphine: The principal alkaloid in opium and the prototype opiate analgesic and narcotic. Morphine has widespread effects in the central nervous system and on smooth muscle. [NIH]

Nephrotoxic: Toxic or destructive to kidney cells. [EU]

Neural: 1. pertaining to a nerve or to the nerves. 2. situated in the region of the spinal axis, as the neutral arch. [EU]

Neuronal: Pertaining to a neuron or neurons (= conducting cells of the nervous system). [EU]

Neurons: The basic cellular units of nervous tissue. Each neuron consists of a body, an axon, and dendrites. Their purpose is to receive, conduct, and transmit impulses in the nervous system. [NIH]

Nicotine: Nicotine is highly toxic alkaloid. It is the prototypical agonist at nicotinic cholinergic receptors where it dramatically stimulates neurons and ultimately blocks synaptic transmission. Nicotine is also important medically because of its presence in tobacco smoke. [NIH]

Nosocomial: Pertaining to or originating in the hospital, said of an infection not present or incubating prior to admittance to the hospital, but generally occurring 72 hours after admittance; the term is usually used to refer to patient disease, but hospital personnel may also acquire nosocomial infection. [EU]

Paralysis: Loss or impairment of motor function in a part due to lesion of the neural or muscular mechanism; also by analogy, impairment of sensory function (sensory paralysis). In addition to the types named below, paralysis is further distinguished as traumatic, syphilitic, toxic, etc., according to its cause; or as obturator, ulnar, etc., according to the nerve part, or muscle specially affected. [EU]

Pathogenesis: The cellular events and reactions that occur in the development of disease. [NIH]

Pharmacokinetics: The action of drugs in the body over a period of time, including the processes of absorption, distribution, localization in tissues, biotransformation, and excretion. [EU]

Phenotype: The entire physical, biochemical, and physiological makeup of an individual as determined by his or her genes and by the environment in the broad sense. [NIH]

Physiologic: Normal; not pathologic; characteristic of or conforming to the normal functioning or state of the body or a tissue or organ; physiological. [EU]

Postnatal: Occurring after birth, with reference to the newborn. [EU]

Proteins: Polymers of amino acids linked by peptide bonds. The specific sequence of amino acids determines the shape and function of the protein. [NIH]

Psoriasis: A common genetically determined, chronic, inflammatory skin disease characterized by rounded erythematous, dry, scaling patches. The lesions have a predilection for nails, scalp, genitalia, extensor surfaces, and the lumbosacral region. Accelerated epidermopoiesis is considered to be the fundamental pathologic feature in psoriasis. [NIH]

Reactivation: The restoration of activity to something that has been inactivated. [EU]

Receptor: 1. a molecular structure within a cell or on the surface characterized by (1) selective binding of a specific substance and (2) a specific physiologic effect that accompanies the binding, e.g., cell-surface receptors for peptide hormones, neurotransmitters, antigens, complement fragments, and immunoglobulins and cytoplasmic receptors for steroid hormones. 2. a sensory nerve terminal that responds to stimuli of various kinds. [EU]

Refractory: Not readily yielding to treatment. [EU]

Salmonella: A genus of gram-negative, facultatively anaerobic, rod-shaped bacteria that utilizes citrate as a sole carbon source. It is pathogenic for humans, causing enteric fevers, gastroenteritis, and bacteremia. Food poisoning is the most common clinical manifestation. Organisms within this genus are separated on the basis of antigenic characteristics, sugar fermentation patterns, and bacteriophage susceptibility. [NIH]

Sclerosis: A induration, or hardening; especially hardening of a part from inflammation and in diseases of the interstitial substance. The term is used chiefly for such a hardening of the nervous system due to hyperplasia of the connective tissue or to designate hardening of the blood vessels. [EU]

Sepsis: The presence of disease-causing organisms or their toxins in the blood. [NIH]

Serum: The clear portion of any body fluid; the clear fluid moistening serous membranes. 2. blood serum; the clear liquid that separates from blood on clotting. 3. immune serum; blood serum from an immunized animal used for passive immunization; an antiserum; antitoxin, or antivenin. [EU]

Stimulant: 1. producing stimulation; especially producing stimulation by causing tension on muscle fibre through the nervous tissue. 2. an agent or remedy that produces stimulation. [EU]

Stroke: Sudden loss of function of part of the brain because of loss of blood flow. Stroke may be caused by a clot (thrombosis) or rupture (hemorrhage) of a blood vessel to the brain. [NIH]

Subacute: Somewhat acute; between acute and chronic. [EU]

Superinfection: A new infection complicating the course of antimicrobial therapy of an existing infectious process, and resulting from invasion by bacteria or fungi resistant to the drug(s) in use. It may occur at the site of the original infection or at a remote site. [EU]

Suppressive: Tending to suppress : effecting suppression; specifically : serving to suppress activity, function, symptoms. [EU]

Synaptic: Pertaining to or affecting a synapse (= site of functional apposition between neurons, at which an impulse is transmitted from one neuron to another by electrical or chemical means); pertaining to synapsis (= pairing off in point-for-point association of homologous chromosomes from the male and female pronuclei during the early prophase of meiosis). [EU]

Synergistic: Acting together; enhancing the effect of another force or agent. [EU]

Thrombosis: The formation, development, or presence of a thrombus. [EU]

Tuberculosis: Any of the infectious diseases of man and other animals caused by species of mycobacterium. [NIH]

Uterus: The hollow muscular organ in female mammals in which the fertilized ovum normally becomes embedded and in which the developing embryo and fetus is nourished. In the nongravid human, it is a pear-shaped structure; about 3 inches in length, consisting of a body, fundus, isthmus, and cervix. Its cavity opens into the vagina below, and into the uterine tube on either side at the cornu. It is supported by direct attachment to the vagina and by indirect attachment to various other nearby pelvic structures. Called also metra. [EU]

Vaccination: The introduction of vaccine into the body for the purpose of inducing immunity. Coined originally to apply to the injection of smallpox vaccine, the term has come to mean any immunizing procedure in which vaccine is injected. [EU]

Vaccine: A suspension of attenuated or killed microorganisms (bacteria, viruses, or rickettsiae), administered for the prevention, amelioration or treatment of infectious diseases. [EU]

Vascular: Pertaining to blood vessels or indicative of a copious blood supply. [EU]

Viremia: The presence of viruses in the blood. [NIH]

Viruses: Minute infectious agents whose genomes are composed of DNA or RNA, but not both. They are characterized by a lack of independent metabolism and the inability to replicate outside living host cells. [NIH]

Withdrawal: 1. a pathological retreat from interpersonal contact and social involvement, as may occur in schizophrenia, depression, or schizoid avoidant and schizotypal personality disorders. 2. (DSM III-R) a substance-specific organic brain syndrome that follows the cessation of use or reduction in intake of a psychoactive substance that had been regularly used to induce a state of intoxication. [EU]

CHAPTER 5. PATENTS ON IMMUNE THROMBOCYTOPENIC PURPURA

Overview

You can learn about innovations relating to immune thrombocytopenic purpura by reading recent patents and patent applications. Patents can be physical innovations (e.g. chemicals, pharmaceuticals, medical equipment) or processes (e.g. treatments or diagnostic procedures). The United States Patent and Trademark Office defines a patent as a grant of a property right to the inventor, issued by the Patent and Trademark Office.[25] Patents, therefore, are intellectual property. For the United States, the term of a new patent is 20 years from the date when the patent application was filed. If the inventor wishes to receive economic benefits, it is likely that the invention will become commercially available to patients with immune thrombocytopenic purpura within 20 years of the initial filing. It is important to understand, therefore, that an inventor's patent does not indicate that a product or service is or will be commercially available to patients with immune thrombocytopenic purpura. The patent implies only that the inventor has "the right to exclude others from making, using, offering for sale, or selling" the invention in the United States. While this relates to U.S. patents, similar rules govern foreign patents.

In this chapter, we show you how to locate information on patents and their inventors. If you find a patent that is particularly interesting to you, contact the inventor or the assignee for further information.

---

[25]Adapted from The U. S. Patent and Trademark Office:
http://www.uspto.gov/web/offices/pac/doc/general/whatis.htm.

Patents on Immune Thrombocytopenic Purpura

By performing a patent search focusing on immune thrombocytopenic purpura, you can obtain information such as the title of the invention, the names of the inventor(s), the assignee(s) or the company that owns or controls the patent, a short abstract that summarizes the patent, and a few excerpts from the description of the patent. The abstract of a patent tends to be more technical in nature, while the description is often written for the public. Full patent descriptions contain much more information than is presented here (e.g. claims, references, figures, diagrams, etc.). We will tell you how to obtain this information later in the chapter. The following is an example of the type of information that you can expect to obtain from a patent search on immune thrombocytopenic purpura:

- **Method for treating patients suffering from immune thrombocytopenic purpura**

  Inventor(s): Jones; Frank R. (Edmonds, WA), Balint, Jr.; Joseph P. (Seattle, WA), Snyder; Harry W. (Edmonds, WA), Jones; Frank R. (Edmonds, WA), Balint, Jr.; Joseph P. (Seattle, WA), Snyder; Harry W. (Edmonds, WA)

  Assignee(s): Cypress Bioscience, Inc. (Seattle, WA), Cypress Bioscience, Inc. (Seattle, WA)

  Patent Number: 5,733,254

  Date filed: May 1, 1995

  Abstract: Immune thrombocytopenic purpura is treated by removal of IgG and circulating immune complexes from the patient's blood. Removal is accomplished by exposing the blood or blood plasma to an immunoadsorbent capable of removing IgG and its complexes. The immunoadsorbent comprises a suitable solid phase coupled to a receptor capable of binding IgG and its complexes, such as protein A. The IgG and its complexes are then removed by the extracorporeal exposure of the patient's blood to the immunoadsorbent, either in a continuous or discontinuous process. In the continuous process, the blood is removed in a steady flow from the patient, separated into its plasma and cellular components, the plasma treated, and the combined cellular components and treated plasma reinfused to the patient. In the discontinuous method, a small volume of blood is removed from the patient, the entire volume separated into plasma and cellular components, the plasma treated, and the entire volume of treated plasma returned to the patient, usually after the cellular components have been returned.

Excerpt(s): The present invention relates generally to the treatment of autoimmune disorders by extracorporeal plasma profusion to remove immunoglobulins and immune complexes. More particularly, the present invention relates to the treatment of immune thrombocytopenic purpura (ITP) by continuous or discontinuous plasma profusion using an immunoadsorbent capable of binding immunoglobulins and immune complexes. ... The present invention relates generally to the treatment of autoimmune disorders by extracorporeal plasma profusion to remove immunoglobulins and immune complexes. More particularly, the present invention relates to the treatment of immune thrombocytopenic purpura (ITP) by continuous or discontinuous plasma profusion using an immunoadsorbent capable of binding immunoglobulins and immune complexes. ... Immune thrombocytopenic purpura (also referred to as idiopathic thrombocytopenic purpura) is a condition characterized by the appearance of lesions resulting from hemorrhage into the skin. ITP occurs in both and acute and chronic forms, and in both forms there are normal or increased numbers of megakaryocytes in the bone marrow, shortened platelet survival time, the presence of bound anti-platelet antibody, and the absence of lymphadenopathy. ... Immune thrombocytopenic purpura (also referred to as idiopathic thrombocytopenic purpura) is a condition characterized by the appearance of lesions resulting from hemorrhage into the skin. ITP occurs in both and acute and chronic forms, and in both forms there are normal or increased numbers of megakaryocytes in the bone marrow, shortened platelet survival time, the presence of bound anti-platelet antibody, and the absence of lymphadenopathy. ... Multiple cases of immune thrombocytopenic purpura have been documented among sexually active homosexual males. See, Abrams et al. (1983) Blood:62:108a, and Karpatkin (1985) Ann. N.Y. Acad. Sci. 437:58. Deposition on platelets of either immune complexes or platelet-specific antibodies appears to be a causative factor in the disease Walsh et al. (1984) N. Eng. J. Med. 311:635. ... Multiple cases of immune thrombocytopenic purpura have been documented among sexually active homosexual males. See, Abrams et al. (1983) Blood:62:108a, and Karpatkin (1985) Ann. N.Y. Acad. Sci. 437:58. Deposition on platelets of either immune complexes or platelet-specific antibodies appears to be a causative factor in the disease Walsh et al. (1984) N. Eng. J. Med. 311:635.

Web site: http://www.delphion.com/details?pn=US05733254__

- **Methods and compositions for diagnosing chronic immune** thrombocytopenic purpura

Inventor(s): McMillan; Robert (Del Mar, CA), Ginsberg; Mark H. (San Diego, CA), Plow; Edward F. (Solon, OH), McMillan; Robert (Del Mar, CA), Ginsberg; Mark H. (San Diego, CA), Plow; Edward F. (Solon, OH)

Assignee(s): The Scripps Research Institute (La Jolla, CA), The Scripps Research Institute (La Jolla, CA)

Patent Number: 5,399,481

Date filed: December 29, 1992

Abstract: The present invention discloses polypeptides consisting essentially of an amino acid residue sequence corresponding to a formula selected from the group consisting of: Tyr-His-Asp-Arg-Lys-Glu-Phe-Ala-Lys-Phe-Glu-Glu-Glu-Arg-Ala-Arg-Ala-Lys-Tr p-Asp-Thr-Ala-Asn-Asn (SEQ ID NO 1); Ala-Asn-Asn-Pro-Leu-Tyr-Lys-Glu-Ala-Thr-Ser-Thr-Phe-Thr-Asn-Ile-Thr-Tyr-Ar g-Gly-Thr (SEQ ID NO 2); Ile-His-Asp-Arg-Lys-Glu-Phe-Ala-Lys-Phe-Glu-Glu-Glu-Arg-Ala-Arg-Ala-Lys-Tr p-Asp-Thr-Ala-Asn-Asn-Pro-Leu-Tyr-Lys-Glu-Ala-Thr-Ser-Thr-Phe-Thr-Asn-Ile-T hr-Tyr-Arg-Gly-Thr (SEQ ID NO 4); and Gly-Pro-Asp-Ile-Leu-Val-Val-Leu-Leu-Ser-Val-Met-Gly-Ala-Ile-Leu-Leu-Thr-Gl y-Leu-Ala-Ala-Leu-Leu-Ile-Trp-Lys-Leu-Leu-Ile-Thr-Ile-His-Asp-Arg-Lys-Glu-P he-Ala-Lys-Phe-Glu-Glu-Glu-Arg-Ala-Arg-Ala-Lys-Trp-Asp-Thr-Ala-Asn-Asn-Pro- Leu-Tyr-Lys-Glu-Ala-Thr-Ser-Thr-Phe-Thr-Asn-Ile-Thr-Tyr-Arg-Gly-Thr (SEQ ID NO 5), as well as diagnostic kits including same. The present invention also discloses methods for determining the presence of anti-GPIIIa autoantibodies in a vascular fluid sample, which autoantibodies are indicative of chronic immune thrombocytopenic purpura in a patient.

Excerpt(s): The present invention relates to polypeptides useful in detecting anti-GPIIIa autoantibodies indicative of chronic immune thrombocytopenic purpura. ... The present invention relates to polypeptides useful in detecting anti-GPIIIa autoantibodies indicative of chronic immune thrombocytopenic purpura. ... Chronic immune thrombocytopenic purpura (ITP) is an autoimmune disorder characterized by thrombocytopenia due to the production of antiplatelet autoantibodies which result in platelet destruction by the reticuloendothelial system or inhibition of platelet production (McMillan, N. Engl. J. Med., 304:1135-1147, 1981; Kelton et al., Semin. Thromb. Haemost., 8:83-104, 1982). Autoantibody from approximately three-fourths of these patients is known to react with the membrane glycoprotein (GP) complexes --GPIIb/IIIa or GPIb/IX (van Leeuwen et al., Blood, 59:23-26, 1982; Woods et al., Blood, 63:368-375, 1984; Woods et al., Blood, 64:156-160, 1984; Beardsley et al., J. Clin. Invest., 74:1701-1707, 1984; McMillan et al., Blood, 70:1040-1045, 1987); of these, some have been shown to bind to GPIIIa (Beardsley et al., J. Clin. Invest., 74:1701-1707, 1984). However, little information is available on the precise location of epitopes on GPIIIa. A recent abstract by Kekomaki et al. showed that plasma from one ITP patient, which reacted with GPIIIa by immunoblotting, bound to a 60,000 dalton GPIIIa fragment resulting from chymotrypsin digestion (Kekomaki et al., Blood, 74:91, 1989). ... Chronic immune thrombocytopenic purpura (ITP) is an autoimmune disorder characterized by thrombocytopenia due to the production of antiplatelet autoantibodies which result in platelet destruction by the reticuloendothelial system or inhibition of platelet production (McMillan, N. Engl. J. Med., 304:1135-1147, 1981; Kelton et al., Semin. Thromb. Haemost., 8:83-104, 1982). Autoantibody from approximately three-fourths of these patients is known to react with the membrane glycoprotein (GP) complexes --GPIIb/IIIa or GPIb/IX (van Leeuwen et al., Blood, 59:23-26, 1982; Woods et al., Blood, 63:368-375, 1984; Woods et al., Blood, 64:156-160, 1984; Beardsley et al., J. Clin. Invest., 74:1701-1707, 1984; McMillan et al., Blood, 70:1040-1045, 1987); of these, some have been shown to bind to GPIIIa (Beardsley et al., J. Clin. Invest., 74:1701-1707, 1984). However, little information is available on the precise location of epitopes on GPIIIa. A recent abstract by Kekomaki et al. showed that plasma from one ITP patient, which reacted with GPIIIa by immunoblotting, bound to a 60,000 dalton GPIIIa fragment resulting from chymotrypsin digestion (Kekomaki et al., Blood, 74:91, 1989). ... The present invention further contemplates a method for determining the presence of anti-GPIIIa autoantibodies in a vascular fluid sample, said autoantibodies being indicative of chronic immune thrombocytopenic purpura in a patient. The method comprises admixing a vascular fluid sample from a patient with a polypeptide of this invention to form an immunoreaction admixture. The admixture thus formed is maintained under biological assay conditions for a period of time sufficient to form an immunoreaction product containing the polypeptide. The presence of the immunoreaction product, and thereby the presence of said anti-GPIIIa autoantibodies is then determined. ... The present invention further contemplates a method for determining the presence of anti-GPIIIa autoantibodies in a vascular fluid sample, said autoantibodies being indicative of chronic immune thrombocytopenic purpura in a patient. The method comprises admixing a vascular fluid sample from a patient with a polypeptide of this invention to form an immunoreaction admixture. The admixture thus formed is maintained under biological assay conditions for a period of time sufficient to form an immunoreaction product containing the polypeptide. The presence of the immunoreaction product, and thereby the presence of said anti-GPIIIa autoantibodies is then determined.

Web site: http://www.delphion.com/details?pn=US05399481__

Patent Applications on Immune Thrombocytopenic Purpura

As of December 2000, U.S. patent applications are open to public viewing.[26] Applications are patent requests which have yet to be granted (the process to achieve a patent can take several years).

Keeping Current

In order to stay informed about patents and patent applications dealing with immune thrombocytopenic purpura, you can access the U.S. Patent Office archive via the Internet at no cost to you. This archive is available at the following Web address: **http://www.uspto.gov/main/patents.htm**. Under "Services," click on "Search Patents." You will see two broad options: (1) Patent Grants, and (2) Patent Applications. To see a list of granted patents, perform the following steps: Under "Patent Grants," click "Quick Search." Then, type "immune thrombocytopenic purpura" (or synonyms) into the "Term 1" box. After clicking on the search button, scroll down to see the various patents which have been granted to date on immune thrombocytopenic purpura. You can also use this procedure to view pending patent applications concerning immune thrombocytopenic purpura. Simply go back to **http://www.uspto.gov/main/patents.htm**. Under "Services," click on "Search Patents." Select "Quick Search" under "Patent Applications." Then proceed with the steps listed above.

Vocabulary Builder

Chymotrypsin: A serine endopeptidase secreted by the pancreas as its zymogen, chymotrypsinogen and carried in the pancreatic juice to the duodenum where it is activated by trypsin. It selectively cleaves aromatic amino acids on the carboxyl side. [NIH]

Megakaryocytes: Very large bone marrow cells which release mature blood platelets. [NIH]

---

[26] This has been a common practice outside the United States prior to December 2000.

CHAPTER 6. BOOKS ON IMMUNE THROMBOCYTOPENIC PURPURA

Overview

This chapter provides bibliographic book references relating to immune thrombocytopenic purpura. You have many options to locate books on immune thrombocytopenic purpura. The simplest method is to go to your local bookseller and inquire about titles that they have in stock or can special order for you. Some patients, however, feel uncomfortable approaching their local booksellers and prefer online sources (e.g. **www.amazon.com** and **www.bn.com**). In addition to online booksellers, excellent sources for book titles on immune thrombocytopenic purpura include the Combined Health Information Database and the National Library of Medicine. Once you have found a title that interests you, visit your local public or medical library to see if it is available for loan.

The National Library of Medicine Book Index

The National Library of Medicine at the National Institutes of Health has a massive database of books published on healthcare and biomedicine. Go to the following Internet site, **http://locatorplus.gov/**, and then select "Search LOCATORplus." Once you are in the search area, simply type "immune thrombocytopenic purpura" (or synonyms) into the search box, and select "books only." From there, results can be sorted by publication date, author, or relevance. The following was recently catalogued by the National Library of Medicine:[27]

---

[27] In addition to LOCATORPlus, in collaboration with authors and publishers, the National Center for Biotechnology Information (NCBI) is adapting biomedical books for the Web. The

- **Activating and inhibitory immunoglobulin-like receptors.**   Author: M.D. Cooper, T. Takai, J.V. Ravetch, (eds.); Year: 2001; Tokyo; New York: Springer, c2001; ISBN: 4431702970 (hard cover: alk. paper) http://www.amazon.com/exec/obidos/ASIN/4431702970/icongroupin terna

- **Annual Congress of the British Society for Immunology: 5-8 December 2000, Harrogate, UK: abstracts.**   Author: [editor, Mike Kemeny; associate editors, John Gordon ... et al.]; Year: 2000; Oxford, UK: Blackwell Science, c2000

- **Basic immunology: functions and disorders of the immune system.** Author: Abul K. Abbas, Andrew H. Lichtman; illustrated by David L. Baker and Alexandra Baker; Year: 2001; Philadelphia: W.B. Saunders Co., c2001; ISBN: 0721693164 http://www.amazon.com/exec/obidos/ASIN/0721693164/icongroupin terna

- **Blackwell's underground clinical vignettes. Pediatrics.**   Author: Vikas Bhushan ... [et al.]; Year: 2002; Malden, Mass.: Blackwell Science, c2002; ISBN: 063204571X (pbk) http://www.amazon.com/exec/obidos/ASIN/063204571X/icongroupi nterna

- **Chronic fatigue syndrome and the body's immune defense system.** Author: Roberto Patarca-Montero; Year: 2001; New York: Haworth Medical Press, c2001; ISBN: 0789015293 (hard: alk. paper) http://www.amazon.com/exec/obidos/ASIN/0789015293/icongroupin terna

- **Clinical immunology: principles and practice.**   Author: edited by Robert R. Rich ... [et al.]; Year: 2001; London New York: Mosby, 2001; ISBN: 0723431612 (set) http://www.amazon.com/exec/obidos/ASIN/0723431612/icongroupin terna

- **Collagen diseases: including systemic lupus erythematosus, polyarteritis, dermatomyositis, systemic scleroderma, thrombotic**

---

books may be accessed in two ways: (1) by searching directly using any search term or phrase (in the same way as the bibliographic database PubMed), or (2) by following the links to PubMed abstracts. Each PubMed abstract has a "Books" button that displays a facsimile of the abstract in which some phrases are hypertext links. These phrases are also found in the books available at NCBI. Click on hyperlinked results in the list of books in which the phrase is found. Currently, the majority of the links are between the books and PubMed. In the future, more links will be created between the books and other types of information, such as gene and protein sequences and macromolecular structures. See **http://www.ncbi.nlm.nih.gov/entrez/query.fcgi?db=Books.**

thrombocytopenic purpura. Author: John H. Talbott and R. Moleres Ferrandis; Year: 1956; New York: Grune & Stratton, 1956

- **Current concepts in experimental gerontology: proceedings of the 12th Weiner Symposium on Experimental Gerontology, Wein, April 23 and 24, 1999.** Author: editors, Carlo Bertoni-Freddari, Hans Niedermüller; Year: 2001; Wien: Facultas Universitätsverlag, [2001?]; ISBN: 3850765253

- **Design principles for the immune system and other distributed autonomous systems.** Author: editors, Lee A. Segel, Irun R. Cohen; Year: 2001; Oxford; New York: Oxford University Press, 2001; ISBN: 0195136993 (alk. paper)
  http://www.amazon.com/exec/obidos/ASIN/0195136993/icongroupin terna

- **Diabetic leg: shin spots, purpura, and gangrene.** Author: Folke Lithner, Hans Melin, and Nils Törnblom; Year: 1987; Umeå, Sweden: Dept. of Medicine, Umeå University Hospital, [1987?]; ISBN: 8787161052

- **Hemolytic uremic syndrome and thrombotic thrombocytopenic purpura.** Author: edited by Bernard S. Kaplan, Richard S. Trompeter, Joel L. Moake; Year: 1992; New York: Marcel Dekker, Inc., c1992; ISBN: 0824786637 (alk. paper)
  http://www.amazon.com/exec/obidos/ASIN/0824786637/icongroupin terna

- **Idiopathic thrombocytopenic purpura: proceedings of a workshop.** Author: editor, Paul Imbach; Year: 1987; Chicago: PharmaLibri, 1987; ISBN: 091983910X (pbk.)
  http://www.amazon.com/exec/obidos/ASIN/091983910X/icongroupi nterna

- **IgA mesangial nephropathy.** Author: First International Milano Meeting of Nephrology on IgA Mesangial Nephropathy, Milano, October 3-4, 1983; volume editors, G. D'Amico, L. Minetti, C. Ponticelli; Year: 1984; Basel; New York: Karger, 1984; ISBN: 3805538774
  http://www.amazon.com/exec/obidos/ASIN/3805538774/icongroupin terna

- **Immune mechanisms of pain analgesia.** Author: Halina Machelska, Christoph Stein; Year: 2001; Georgetown, TX: Eurekah.com/Landes Bioscience, c2001; ISBN: 1587060620 (hardcover)
  http://www.amazon.com/exec/obidos/ASIN/1587060620/icongroupin terna

- **Immunology: theoretical & practical concepts in laboratory medicine.** Author: Hannah D. Zane; Year: 2001; Philadelphia: W.B. Saunders, c2001; ISBN: 0721650023

http://www.amazon.com/exec/obidos/ASIN/0721650023/icongroupin
terna

- **Immunology for the boards and wards.** Author: Carlos Ayala, Brad Spellberg; Year: 2001; Malden, Mass.: Blackwell Science, c2001; ISBN: 0632045744
  http://www.amazon.com/exec/obidos/ASIN/0632045744/icongroupin
  terna

- **Immunology, immunopathology, and immunity.** Author: Stewart Sell; contributing author, Edward E. Max; Year: 2001; Washington, D.C.: ASM Press, c2001; ISBN: 1555812023
  http://www.amazon.com/exec/obidos/ASIN/1555812023/icongroupin
  terna

- **Immunology.** Author: [edited by] Ivan Roitt, Jonathan Brostoff, David Male; Year: 2001; Edinburgh; New York: Mosby, 2001; ISBN: 0723431892
  http://www.amazon.com/exec/obidos/ASIN/0723431892/icongroupin
  terna

- **Infectious disease risks associated with exposure to stressful environments.** Author: Richard T. Meehan and Morey Smith, Clarence Sams; Year: 1993; Warrendale, PA: SAE International, 1993

- **Intravenous immunoglobulins in immunodeficiency syndromes and idiopathic thrombocytopenic purpura.** Author: edited by A.H. Waters and A.D.B. Webster; Year: 1985; London: Royal Society of Medicine; Oxford; New York: Distributed by Oxford University Press, 1985; ISBN: 0199220239 (pbk.)
  http://www.amazon.com/exec/obidos/ASIN/0199220239/icongroupin
  terna

- **Medical immunology made memorable.** Author: J. H. L. Playfair and P. M. Lydyard; Year: 2000; Edinburgh; New York: Churchill Livingstone, 2000; ISBN: 0443064296
  http://www.amazon.com/exec/obidos/ASIN/0443064296/icongroupin
  terna

- **Multisystem diseases.** Author: editor, G.R.D. Catto; Year: 1989; Dordrecht; Boston: Kluwer Academic Publishers, c1989; ISBN: 0746200609 (U.S.)
  http://www.amazon.com/exec/obidos/ASIN/0746200609/icongroupin
  terna

- **Observations on megakaryocytopoiesis and thrombocytopoiesis in chronic idiopathic thrombocytopenic purpura.** Author: door Wilhelmus Petrus Maria Breed; Year: 1974; [Meppel?: s.n.], 1974

- **Phylogenetic perspectives on the vertebrate immune system.** Author: edited by Gregory Beck, Manickam Sugumaran, and Edwin L. Cooper;

Year: 2001; New York: Kluwer Academic/Plenum Publishers, c2001;
ISBN: 0306464314

http://www.amazon.com/exec/obidos/ASIN/0306464314/icongroupin
terna

- **Purpuras.** Author: Harrington, William Joseph, 1923-; Year: 1957;
  Chicago, Year Book Publishers, 1957

- **Roitt's essential immunology.** Author: Ivan M. Roitt, Peter J. Delves;
  Year: 2001; Oxford; Malden, MA: Blackwell Science, 2001; ISBN:
  0632059028 (pbk.)

  http://www.amazon.com/exec/obidos/ASIN/0632059028/icongroupin
  terna

- **Studies on platelet survival and platelet production in idiopathic
  thrombocytopenic prupura.** Author: by Ingmar Branehög; Year: 1974;
  Göteborg, [Sweden: s.n.], 1974

- **Study of the megakaryocytes and eosinophils in the bone marrow in
  essential thrombocytopenic purpura and the clinical significance of
  these findings.** Author: Diessner, Grant Roy; Year: 1949; [Minneapolis]
  1949

- **Thrombotic thrombocytopenic purpura.** Author: Leavitt, Clark Thomas,
  1928-; Year: 1958; [Minneapolis] 1958

- **War within us: everyman's guide to infection and immunity.** Author:
  Cedric Mims; Year: 2000; San Diego, CA.: Academic Press, c2000; ISBN:
  0124982514 (alk. paper)

  http://www.amazon.com/exec/obidos/ASIN/0124982514/icongroupin
  terna

Chapters on Immune Thrombocytopenic Purpura

Frequently, immune thrombocytopenic purpura will be discussed within a
book, perhaps within a specific chapter. In order to find chapters that are
specifically dealing with immune thrombocytopenic purpura, an excellent
source of abstracts is the Combined Health Information Database. You will
need to limit your search to book chapters and immune thrombocytopenic
purpura using the "Detailed Search" option. Go directly to the following
hyperlink: **http://chid.nih.gov/detail/detail.html**. To find book chapters, use
the drop boxes at the bottom of the search page where "You may refine your
search by." Select the dates and language you prefer, and the format option
"Book Chapter." By making these selections and typing in "immune
thrombocytopenic purpura" (or synonyms) into the "For these words:" box,
you will only receive results on chapters in books. The following is a typical

result when searching for book chapters on immune thrombocytopenic purpura:

- **Oral Manifestations of HIV Infection and AIDS**

  Source: in Merigan, T.C., Jr.; Bartlett, J.G.; Bolognesi, D., eds. Textbook of AIDS Medicine. 2nd ed. Baltimore, MD: Williams and Wilkins. 1999. p. 521-535.

  Contact: Available from Williams and Wilkins. 351 West Camden Street, Baltimore, MD 21201-2436. (800) 638-0672. Fax (800) 447-8438. E-mail: custserv@wwilkins.com. Website: www.wwilkins.com. PRICE: $155.00. ISBN: 0683302167.

  Summary: This chapter from a textbook of AIDS medicine focuses on the oral manifestations of HIV infection and AIDS. Topics include epidemiology, including the significance of oral manifestations, the prevalence, incidence, and classification of these findings; neoplasms, including Kaposi's sarcoma, lymphoma, and oral cancer; fungal lesions, including oral candidiasis, erythematous candidiasis, pseudomembranous candidiasis, and angular cheilitis; viral lesions, including herpes simplex, varicella zoster virus (VZV), cytomegalovirus, hairy leukoplakia, and papillomavirus lesions; bacterial infections, including periodontal diseases such as gingivitis and necrotizing ulcerative periodontitis; idiopathic or autoimmune lesions, including recurrent aphthous ulcers, HIV-associated salivary gland disease, immune thrombocytopenic purpura, and abnormal pigmentation; the oral complications associated with pediatric HIV infection; and other oral problems associated with HIV infection. For each condition discussed, the authors report symptoms, diagnosis, and basic management strategies, including drug therapy where appropriate. The authors conclude that initial clinical impressions concerning the frequency of oral lesions and their place in the natural history and progression of HIV disease and AIDS have been supported by a substantial number of studies. However, standardized classification schemes, definitions, and diagnostic criteria are far from being applied universally. 12 figures. 1 table. 191 references.

General Home References

In addition to references for immune thrombocytopenic purpura, you may want a general home medical guide that spans all aspects of home healthcare. The following list is a recent sample of such guides (sorted alphabetically by title; hyperlinks provide rankings, information, and reviews at Amazon.com):

- **American College of Physicians Complete Home Medical Guide (with Interactive Human Anatomy CD-ROM)** by David R. Goldmann (Editor), American College of Physicians; Hardcover - 1104 pages, Book & CD-Rom edition (1999), DK Publishing; ISBN: 0789444127;
  http://www.amazon.com/exec/obidos/ASIN/0789444127/icongroupinterna

- **The American Medical Association Guide to Home Caregiving** by the American Medical Association (Editor); Paperback - 256 pages, 1st edition (2001), John Wiley & Sons; ISBN: 0471414093;
  http://www.amazon.com/exec/obidos/ASIN/0471414093/icongroupinterna

- **Anatomica : The Complete Home Medical Reference** by Peter Forrestal (Editor); Hardcover (2000), Book Sales; ISBN: 1740480309;
  http://www.amazon.com/exec/obidos/ASIN/1740480309/icongroupinterna

- **The HarperCollins Illustrated Medical Dictionary : The Complete Home Medical Dictionary** by Ida G. Dox, et al; Paperback - 656 pages, 4th edition (2001), Harper Resource; ISBN: 0062736469;
  http://www.amazon.com/exec/obidos/ASIN/0062736469/icongroupinterna

- **Mayo Clinic Guide to Self-Care: Answers for Everyday Health Problems** by Philip Hagen, M.D. (Editor), et al; Paperback - 279 pages, 2nd edition (December 15, 1999), Kensington Publishing Corp.; ISBN: 0962786578;
  http://www.amazon.com/exec/obidos/ASIN/0962786578/icongroupinterna

- **The Merck Manual of Medical Information: Home Edition (Merck Manual of Medical Information Home Edition (Trade Paper)** by Robert Berkow (Editor), Mark H. Beers, M.D. (Editor); **Paperback** - 1536 pages (2000), Pocket Books; ISBN: 0671027263;
  http://www.amazon.com/exec/obidos/ASIN/0671027263/icongroupinterna

- **What Do You Know About Hematology (Test Your Knowledge Series (Q - 68))** by Jack Rudman; (Paperback - February 1997), National Learning Corporation; ISBN: 083737068X;
  http://www.amazon.com/exec/obidos/ASIN/083737068X/icongroupinterna

Vocabulary Builder

Cheilitis: Inflammation of the lips. It is of various etiologies and degrees of pathology. [NIH]

Contraception: The prevention of conception or impregnation. [EU]

Cytomegalovirus: A genus of the family herpesviridae, subfamily betaherpesvirinae, infecting the salivary glands, liver, spleen, lungs, eyes, and other organs, in which they produce characteristically enlarged cells with intranuclear inclusions. Infection with Cytomegalovirus is also seen as an opportunistic infection in AIDS. [NIH]

Eosinophils: Granular leukocytes with a nucleus that usually has two lobes connected by a slender thread of chromatin, and cytoplasm containing coarse, round granules that are uniform in size and stainable by eosin. [NIH]

Fatigue: The state of weariness following a period of exertion, mental or physical, characterized by a decreased capacity for work and reduced efficiency to respond to stimuli. [NIH]

Gingivitis: Inflammation of the gingivae. Gingivitis associated with bony changes is referred to as periodontitis. Called also oulitis and ulitis. [EU]

Lymphoma: Cancer of the lymph nodes. [NIH]

Neoplasms: New abnormal growth of tissue. Malignant neoplasms show a greater degree of anaplasia and have the properties of invasion and metastasis, compared to benign neoplasms. [NIH]

Nephrology: A subspecialty of internal medicine concerned with the anatomy, physiology, and pathology of the kidney. [NIH]

Nephropathy: Disease of the kidneys. [EU]

Papillomavirus: A genus of papovaviridae causing proliferation of the epithelium, which may lead to malignancy. A wide range of animals are infected including humans, chimpanzees, cattle, rabbits, dogs, and horses. [NIH]

Pigmentation: 1. the deposition of colouring matter; the coloration or discoloration of a part by pigment. 2. coloration, especially abnormally increased coloration, by melanin. [EU]

Prevalence: The number of events, e.g., instances of a given disease or other condition, in a given population at a designated time. When used without qualification, the term usually refers to the situation at specific point in time (point prevalence). Prevalence is a number, not a rate. [NIH]

Sarcoma: A tumour made up of a substance like the embryonic connective tissue; tissue composed of closely packed cells embedded in a fibrillar or homogeneous substance. Sarcomas are often highly malignant. [EU]

CHAPTER 7. MULTIMEDIA ON IMMUNE THROMBOCYTOPENIC PURPURA

Overview

Information on immune thrombocytopenic purpura can come in a variety of formats. Among multimedia sources, video productions, slides, audiotapes, and computer databases are often available. In this chapter, we show you how to keep current on multimedia sources of information on immune thrombocytopenic purpura. We start with sources that have been summarized by federal agencies, and then show you how to find bibliographic information catalogued by the National Library of Medicine. If you see an interesting item, visit your local medical library to check on the availability of the title.

Bibliography: Multimedia on Immune Thrombocytopenic Purpura

The National Library of Medicine is a rich source of information on healthcare-related multimedia productions including slides, computer software, and databases. To access the multimedia database, go to the following Web site: **http://locatorplus.gov/**. Select "Search LOCATORplus." Once in the search area, simply type in immune thrombocytopenic purpura (or synonyms). Then, in the option box provided below the search box, select "Audiovisuals and Computer Files." From here, you can choose to sort results by publication date, author, or relevance. The following multimedia has been indexed on immune thrombocytopenic purpura. For more information, follow the hyperlink indicated:

- **Basic concepts in immunology.**   Source: University of Wisconsin--Madison; Year: 1988; Format: Videorecording; [Madison, Wis.]: The University, [1988]

- **Basic hematology.**   Source: Edward L. Amorosi; Year: 1970; Format: Slide; [New York]: Medcom, c1970

- **Basic hematology.**   Source: Trainex Corporation; Year: 1972; Format: Filmstrip; [Garden Grove, Calif.]: Trainex, c1972

- **Body story. Infiltration by influenza B.**   Source: a presentation of Films for the Humanities & Sciences; a Wall to Wall Television Ltd production for Discovery Channel, Channel Four, and ITEL; Year: 1999; Format: Videorecording; Princeton, N.J.: Films for the Humanities & Sciences, c1999

- **Clinical immunology: principles and practice.**   Source: edited by Robert R. Rich ... ; Year: 2001; Format: Et al; London New York: Mosby, 2001

- **Coagulation.**   Source: [by Elizabeth Hartwell, Alan H. Wu]; Year: 1990; Format: Electronic resource; Chapel Hill, NC: Health Sciences Consortium, [1990]

- **Determination of bleeding and clotting time.**   Source: Department of Pathology [and] Educational Resources Group, University of Missouri-Columbia, Medical Center; Year: 1969; Format: Slide; Columbia, Mo.: The Department, 1969

- **Immune response.**   Source: [presented by] CRM Films; [produced by Sierra Productions]; Year: 1989; Format: Videorecording; San Diego, CA: Sierra Productions, c1989

- **Immunodeficiency : a disease of life.**   Source: [presented by] CRM Films; Sierra Productions; Year: 1989; Format: Videorecording; San Diego, CA: Sierra Productions, c1989

- **Immunology for life scientists: a basic introduction: a student-centered learning approach.**   Source: Lesley-Jane Eales; Year: 1997; Chichester; New York: Wiley, 1997

- **Immunology.**   Source: Ivan Roitt, Jonathan Brostoff, David Male; Year: 2001; Format: Edited by; Edinburgh; New York: Mosby, 2001

- **Immunology.**   Source: Richard M. Hyde; Year: 2000; Format: Edited by; Philadelphia: Lippincott Williams & Wilkins, c2000

- **Influenza.**   Source: a film by Bruno Carrière; [presented by] Films for the Humanities & Sciences; NFB ONF, a coproduction of the National Film Board of Canada, Les Films d'lci, and France 2; Year: 1998; Format: Videorecording; Princeton, N.J.: Films for the Humanities & Sciences, c1998

- **Laparoscopic splenectomy in childhood.** Source: by Thom E. Lobe; American College of Surgeons; Year: 1993; Format: Videorecording; [United States]: T.E. Lobe, c1993

- **Morphology of red blood cells.** Source: Cleveland Clinic Educational Foundation; Year: 1974; Format: Videorecording; Cleveland, Ohio: The Foundation: [for sale by Cleveland Clinic Educational Foundation, Audiovisual Dept., 1974]

- **Mucosal immunity and disease .** Year: 1994; Format: Sound recording; [Bethesda, Md.]: American Gastroenterological Association, [1994]

- **Neonatal immune system : relevance to the pediatrician.** Source: [presented by] Marshfield Video Network, in cooperation with Marshfield Medical Research Foundation, Marshfield Clinic, [and] St. Joseph's Hospital; Year: 1987; Format: Videorecording; Marshfield, WI: The Network, c1987

- **Nutrient effects on the immune system.** Source: produced by UT/TV-Houston, the University of Texas Health Science Center at Houston; Year: 1990; Format: Videorecording; [Houston, Tex.: UT/TV], c1990

- **Pathways of peripheral T-cell tolerance.** Source: [Richard Flavell]; Year: 1996; Format: Sound recording; [Bethesda, Md.: National Institutes of Health, 1996]

- **Pediatric hematology.** Source: Sergio Piomelli, Laurence M. Corash; Year: 1971; Format: Slide; New York: Medcom, c1971

- **Renal biopsy.** Source: Richard R. Lindquist; Year: 1970; Format: Slide; [New York]: Medcom, c1970

- **Rubella.** Source: Center for Disease Control, Bureau of Training, Instructional Systems Division; Year: 1969; Format: Slide; [Atlanta: The Center, 1969?]

- **Self recognition : recent insights into the deepest puzzle in immunology.** Source: [Gustav J. Nossal]; Year: 1993; Format: Sound recording; [Bethesda, Md.: National Institutes of Health, 1993]

- **Splenectomy: indications and technique.** Source: Robert E. Hermann, John D. Battle, James S. Hewlett; [made by Movie Makers, Inc.]; Year: 1967; Format: Motion picture; [Cleveland: Hermann; [Atlanta: for loan by National Medical Audiovisual Center, 1967]

- **Stress : immunologic aspects.** Source: sponsored by the Office of Research on Women's Health, NIH, in collaboration with the Advisory Committee on Women's Health Issues and the Working Group on Health and Beahavior; Year: 1993; Format: Videorecording; Bethesda, Md.: The Office, 1993

- **Thrombocytopenia in pregnancy.** Source: [presented by] the Emory Medical Television Network, Emory University, School of Medicine of the Robert Woodruff Health Sciences Center; Year: 1992; Format: Videorecording; Atlanta, Ga.: The University, c1992

- **Update on the diagnosis and management of purpura.** Source: Warren W. Piette; Year: 1994; Format: Videorecording; Secaucus, N.J.: Network for Continuing Medical Education, 1994

- **What's killing the children?** Source: [presented by] WGBH Boston; a production of the Production Group Inc. in association with WGBH Boston; Year: 1990; Format: Videorecording; [Boston, Mass.]: WGBH Educational Foundation, c1990

Vocabulary Builder

Biopsy: The removal and examination, usually microscopic, of tissue from the living body, performed to establish precise diagnosis. [EU]

Infiltration: The diffusion or accumulation in a tissue or cells of substances not normal to it or in amounts of the normal. Also, the material so accumulated. [EU]

Lobe: A more or less well-defined portion of any organ, especially of the brain, lungs, and glands. Lobes are demarcated by fissures, sulci, connective tissue, and by their shape. [EU]

CHAPTER 8. PHYSICIAN GUIDELINES AND DATABASES

Overview

Doctors and medical researchers rely on a number of information sources to help patients with their conditions. Many will subscribe to journals or newsletters published by their professional associations or refer to specialized textbooks or clinical guides published for the medical profession. In this chapter, we focus on databases and Internet-based guidelines created or written for this professional audience.

NIH Guidelines

For the more common diseases, The National Institutes of Health publish guidelines that are frequently consulted by physicians. Publications are typically written by one or more of the various NIH Institutes. For physician guidelines, commonly referred to as "clinical" or "professional" guidelines, you can visit the following Institutes:

- Office of the Director (OD); guidelines consolidated across agencies available at **http://www.nih.gov/health/consumer/conkey.htm**

- National Institute of General Medical Sciences (NIGMS); fact sheets available at **http://www.nigms.nih.gov/news/facts/**

- National Library of Medicine (NLM); extensive encyclopedia (A.D.A.M., Inc.) with guidelines:
  http://www.nlm.nih.gov/medlineplus/healthtopics.html

- National Heart, Lung, and Blood Institute (NHLBI); guidelines available at **http://www.nhlbi.nih.gov/guidelines/index.htm**

The NHLBI recently recommended the following guidelines and references to physicians treating patients with blood-related conditions:

Sickle Cell Disease Information

- Management and Therapy of Sickle Cell Disease:
  http://www.nhlbi.nih.gov/health/prof/blood/sickle/sick-mt.htm

- Sickle Cell Disease Advisory Committee:
  http://www.nhlbi.nih.gov/meetings/scd/index.htm

Blood Transfusion Safety Information

- Transfusion Alert: Use of Autologous Blood:
  http://www.nhlbi.nih.gov/health/prof/blood/transfusion/logo.htm

- Transfusion Alert: Indications for the Use of Red Blood Cells, Platelets, and Fresh Frozen Plasma:
  http://www.nhlbi.nih.gov/health/prof/blood/transfusion/transfin.htm

Other Blood Information

- Research Agenda on Complications of Hemophilia and Other Bleeding Disorders:
  http://www.nhlbi.nih.gov/health/prof/blood/other/hemophilia/index.htm

- Cooley's Anemia: Progress in Biology and Medicine-1995:
  http://www.nhlbi.nih.gov/health/prof/blood/other/cooleys.htm

- Blood Information for Patients and the General Public:
  http://www.nhlbi.nih.gov/health/public/blood/index.htm

- List of Publications: http://www.nhlbi.nih.gov/health/pubs/index.htm

- Information Center: http://www.nhlbi.nih.gov/health/infoctr/index.htm

- National Cancer Institute (for cancers of the blood):
  http://www.nci.nih.gov/

NIH Databases

In addition to the various Institutes of Health that publish professional guidelines, the NIH has designed a number of databases for professionals.[28] Physician-oriented resources provide a wide variety of information related to the biomedical and health sciences, both past and present. The format of these resources varies. Searchable databases, bibliographic citations, full text articles (when available), archival collections, and images are all available. The following are referenced by the National Library of Medicine:[29]

- **Bioethics:** Access to published literature on the ethical, legal and public policy issues surrounding healthcare and biomedical research. This information is provided in conjunction with the Kennedy Institute of Ethics located at Georgetown University, Washington, D.C.: **http://www.nlm.nih.gov/databases/databases_bioethics.html**

- **HIV/AIDS Resources:** Describes various links and databases dedicated to HIV/AIDS research: **http://www.nlm.nih.gov/pubs/factsheets/aidsinfs.html**

- **NLM Online Exhibitions:** Describes "Exhibitions in the History of Medicine": **http://www.nlm.nih.gov/exhibition/exhibition.html**. Additional resources for historical scholarship in medicine: **http://www.nlm.nih.gov/hmd/hmd.html**

- **Biotechnology Information:** Access to public databases. The National Center for Biotechnology Information conducts research in computational biology, develops software tools for analyzing genome data, and disseminates biomedical information for the better understanding of molecular processes affecting human health and disease: **http://www.ncbi.nlm.nih.gov/**

- **Population Information:** The National Library of Medicine provides access to worldwide coverage of population, family planning, and related health issues, including family planning technology and programs, fertility, and population law and policy: **http://www.nlm.nih.gov/databases/databases_population.html**

- **Cancer Information:** Access to caner-oriented databases: **http://www.nlm.nih.gov/databases/databases_cancer.html**

---

[28] Remember, for the general public, the National Library of Medicine recommends the databases referenced in MEDLINE*plus* (**http://medlineplus.gov/** or **http://www.nlm.nih.gov/medlineplus/databases.html**).

[29] See http://www.nlm.nih.gov/databases/databases.html.

- **Profiles in Science:** Offering the archival collections of prominent twentieth-century biomedical scientists to the public through modern digital technology: **http://www.profiles.nlm.nih.gov/**

- **Chemical Information:** Provides links to various chemical databases and references: **http://sis.nlm.nih.gov/Chem/ChemMain.html**

- **Clinical Alerts:** Reports the release of findings from the NIH-funded clinical trials where such release could significantly affect morbidity and mortality: **http://www.nlm.nih.gov/databases/alerts/clinical_alerts.html**

- **Space Life Sciences:** Provides links and information to space-based research (including NASA): **http://www.nlm.nih.gov/databases/databases_space.html**

- **MEDLINE:** Bibliographic database covering the fields of medicine, nursing, dentistry, veterinary medicine, the healthcare system, and the pre-clinical sciences: **http://www.nlm.nih.gov/databases/databases_medline.html**

- **Toxicology and Environmental Health Information (TOXNET):** Databases covering toxicology and environmental health: **http://sis.nlm.nih.gov/Tox/ToxMain.html**

- **Visible Human Interface:** Anatomically detailed, three-dimensional representations of normal male and female human bodies: **http://www.nlm.nih.gov/research/visible/visible_human.html**

While all of the above references may be of interest to physicians who study and treat immune thrombocytopenic purpura, the following are particularly noteworthy.

The NLM Gateway[30]

The NLM (National Library of Medicine) Gateway is a Web-based system that lets users search simultaneously in multiple retrieval systems at the U.S. National Library of Medicine (NLM). It allows users of NLM services to initiate searches from one Web interface, providing "one-stop searching" for many of NLM's information resources or databases.[31] One target audience for the Gateway is the Internet user who is new to NLM's online resources and does not know what information is available or how best to search for it.

---

30 Adapted from NLM: **http://gateway.nlm.nih.gov/gw/Cmd?Overview.x**.
31 The NLM Gateway is currently being developed by the Lister Hill National Center for Biomedical Communications (LHNCBC) at the National Library of Medicine (NLM) of the National Institutes of Health (NIH).

This audience may include physicians and other healthcare providers, researchers, librarians, students, and, increasingly, patients, their families, and the public.[32] To use the NLM Gateway, simply go to the search site at **http://gateway.nlm.nih.gov/gw/Cmd**. Type "immune thrombocytopenic purpura" (or synonyms) into the search box and click "Search." The results will be presented in a tabular form, indicating the number of references in each database category.

Results Summary

Category	Items Found
Journal Articles	1501
Books / Periodicals / Audio Visual	4
Consumer Health	11
Meeting Abstracts	13
Other Collections	0
Total	1529

HSTAT[33]

HSTAT is a free, Web-based resource that provides access to full-text documents used in healthcare decision-making.[34] HSTAT's audience includes healthcare providers, health service researchers, policy makers, insurance companies, consumers, and the information professionals who serve these groups. HSTAT provides access to a wide variety of publications, including clinical practice guidelines, quick-reference guides for clinicians, consumer health brochures, evidence reports and technology assessments from the Agency for Healthcare Research and Quality (AHRQ), as well as

---

[32] Other users may find the Gateway useful for an overall search of NLM's information resources. Some searchers may locate what they need immediately, while others will utilize the Gateway as an adjunct tool to other NLM search services such as PubMed® and MEDLINEplus®. The Gateway connects users with multiple NLM retrieval systems while also providing a search interface for its own collections. These collections include various types of information that do not logically belong in PubMed, LOCATORplus, or other established NLM retrieval systems (e.g., meeting announcements and pre-1966 journal citations). The Gateway will provide access to the information found in an increasing number of NLM retrieval systems in several phases.

[33] Adapted from HSTAT: **http://www.nlm.nih.gov/pubs/factsheets/hstat.html**

[34] The HSTAT URL is **http://hstat.nlm.nih.gov/**.

AHRQ's Put Prevention Into Practice.[35] Simply search by "immune thrombocytopenic purpura" (or synonyms) at the following Web site: **http://text.nlm.nih.gov**.

Coffee Break: Tutorials for Biologists[36]

Some patients may wish to have access to a general healthcare site that takes a scientific view of the news and covers recent breakthroughs in biology that may one day assist physicians in developing treatments. To this end, we recommend "Coffee Break," a collection of short reports on recent biological discoveries. Each report incorporates interactive tutorials that demonstrate how bioinformatics tools are used as a part of the research process. Currently, all Coffee Breaks are written by NCBI staff.[37] Each report is about 400 words and is usually based on a discovery reported in one or more articles from recently published, peer-reviewed literature.[38] This site has new articles every few weeks, so it can be considered an online magazine of sorts, and intended for general background information. You can access the Coffee Break Web site at **http://www.ncbi.nlm.nih.gov/Coffeebreak/**.

---

[35] Other important documents in HSTAT include: the National Institutes of Health (NIH) Consensus Conference Reports and Technology Assessment Reports; the HIV/AIDS Treatment Information Service (ATIS) resource documents; the Substance Abuse and Mental Health Services Administration's Center for Substance Abuse Treatment (SAMHSA/CSAT) Treatment Improvement Protocols (TIP) and Center for Substance Abuse Prevention (SAMHSA/CSAP) Prevention Enhancement Protocols System (PEPS); the Public Health Service (PHS) Preventive Services Task Force's *Guide to Clinical Preventive Services*; the independent, nonfederal Task Force on Community Services *Guide to Community Preventive Services*; and the Health Technology Advisory Committee (HTAC) of the Minnesota Health Care Commission (MHCC) health technology evaluations.

[36] Adapted from **http://www.ncbi.nlm.nih.gov/Coffeebreak/Archive/FAQ.html**

[37] The figure that accompanies each article is frequently supplied by an expert external to NCBI, in which case the source of the figure is cited. The result is an interactive tutorial that tells a biological story.

[38] After a brief introduction that sets the work described into a broader context, the report focuses on how a molecular understanding can provide explanations of observed biology and lead to therapies for diseases. Each vignette is accompanied by a figure and hypertext links that lead to a series of pages that interactively show how NCBI tools and resources are used in the research process.

Other Commercial Databases

In addition to resources maintained by official agencies, other databases exist that are commercial ventures addressing medical professionals. Here are a few examples that may interest you:

- **CliniWeb International:** Index and table of contents to selected clinical information on the Internet; see **http://www.ohsu.edu/cliniweb/**.

- **Image Engine:** Multimedia electronic medical record system that integrates a wide range of digitized clinical images with textual data stored in the University of Pittsburgh Medical Center's MARS electronic medical record system; see the following Web site: **http://www.cml.upmc.edu/cml/imageengine/imageEngine.html**.

- **Medical World Search:** Searches full text from thousands of selected medical sites on the Internet; see **http://www.mwsearch.com/**.

- **MedWeaver:** Prototype system that allows users to search differential diagnoses for any list of signs and symptoms, to search medical literature, and to explore relevant Web sites; see **http://www.med.virginia.edu/~wmd4n/medweaver.html**.

- **Metaphrase:** Middleware component intended for use by both caregivers and medical records personnel. It converts the informal language generally used by caregivers into terms from formal, controlled vocabularies; see **http://www.lexical.com/Metaphrase.html**.

The Genome Project and Immune Thrombocytopenic Purpura

With all the discussion in the press about the Human Genome Project, it is only natural that physicians, researchers, and patients want to know about how human genes relate to immune thrombocytopenic purpura. In the following section, we will discuss databases and references used by physicians and scientists who work in this area.

Online Mendelian Inheritance in Man (OMIM)

The Online Mendelian Inheritance in Man (OMIM) database is a catalog of human genes and genetic disorders authored and edited by Dr. Victor A. McKusick and his colleagues at Johns Hopkins and elsewhere. OMIM was developed for the World Wide Web by the National Center for

Biotechnology Information (NCBI).[39] The database contains textual information, pictures, and reference information. It also contains copious links to NCBI's Entrez database of MEDLINE articles and sequence information.

Go to **http://www.ncbi.nlm.nih.gov/Omim/searchomim.html** to search the database. Type "immune thrombocytopenic purpura" (or synonyms) in the search box, and click "Submit Search." If too many results appear, you can narrow the search by adding the word "clinical." Each report will have additional links to related research and databases. By following these links, especially the link titled "Database Links," you will be exposed to numerous specialized databases that are largely used by the scientific community. These databases are overly technical and seldom used by the general public, but offer an abundance of information. The following is an example of the results you can obtain from the OMIM for immune thrombocytopenic purpura:

- **Adenosine Deaminase**
  Web site: http://www.ncbi.nlm.nih.gov/htbin-post/Omim/dispmim?102700

- **Autoimmune Diseases**
  Web site: http://www.ncbi.nlm.nih.gov/htbin-post/Omim/dispmim?109100

- **Autoimmune Lymphoproliferative Syndrome, Type Ii**
  Web site: http://www.ncbi.nlm.nih.gov/htbin-post/Omim/dispmim?603909

- **Cd36 Antigen**
  Web site: http://www.ncbi.nlm.nih.gov/htbin-post/Omim/dispmim?173510

- **Digeorge Syndrome**
  Web site: http://www.ncbi.nlm.nih.gov/htbin-post/Omim/dispmim?188400

- **Hemolytic-uremic Syndrome**
  Web site: http://www.ncbi.nlm.nih.gov/htbin-post/Omim/dispmim?235400

---

[39] Adapted from **http://www.ncbi.nlm.nih.gov/**. Established in 1988 as a national resource for molecular biology information, NCBI creates public databases, conducts research in computational biology, develops software tools for analyzing genome data, and disseminates biomedical information--all for the better understanding of molecular processes affecting human health and disease.

- **Integrin, Beta-3**
  Web site: http://www.ncbi.nlm.nih.gov/htbin-post/Omim/dispmim?173470

- **Kabuki Syndrome**
  Web site: http://www.ncbi.nlm.nih.gov/htbin-post/Omim/dispmim?147920

- **Lupus Erythematosus, Systemic**
  Web site: http://www.ncbi.nlm.nih.gov/htbin-post/Omim/dispmim?152700

- **Reticulosis, Familial Histiocytic**
  Web site: http://www.ncbi.nlm.nih.gov/htbin-post/Omim/dispmim?267700

Genes and Disease (NCBI - Map)

The Genes and Disease database is produced by the National Center for Biotechnology Information of the National Library of Medicine at the National Institutes of Health. This Web site categorizes each disorder by the system of the body associated with it. Go to **http://www.ncbi.nlm.nih.gov/disease/**, and browse the system pages to have a full view of important conditions linked to human genes. Since this site is regularly updated, you may wish to re-visit it from time to time. The following systems and associated disorders are addressed:

- **Immune System:** Fights invaders.
  Examples: Asthma, autoimmune polyglandular syndrome, Crohn's disease, DiGeorge syndrome, familial Mediterranean fever, immunodeficiency with Hyper-IgM, severe combined immunodeficiency.
  Web site: **http://www.ncbi.nlm.nih.gov/disease/Immune.html**

- **Metabolism:** Food and energy.
  Examples: Adreno-leukodystrophy, Atherosclerosis, Best disease, Gaucher disease, Glucose galactose malabsorption, Gyrate atrophy, Juvenile onset diabetes, Obesity, Paroxysmal nocturnal hemoglobinuria, Phenylketonuria, Refsum disease, Tangier disease, Tay-Sachs disease.
  Web site: **http://www.ncbi.nlm.nih.gov/disease/Metabolism.html**

- **Muscle and Bone:** Movement and growth.
  Examples: Duchenne muscular dystrophy, Ellis-van Creveld syndrome, Marfan syndrome, myotonic dystrophy, spinal muscular atrophy.
  Web site: **http://www.ncbi.nlm.nih.gov/disease/Muscle.html**

- **Transporters:** Pumps and channels.
  Examples: Cystic Fibrosis, deafness, diastrophic dysplasia, Hemophilia A, long-QT syndrome, Menkes syndrome, Pendred syndrome, polycystic kidney disease, sickle cell anemia, Wilson's disease, Zellweger syndrome.
  Web site: **http://www.ncbi.nlm.nih.gov/disease/Transporters.html**

Entrez

Entrez is a search and retrieval system that integrates several linked databases at the National Center for Biotechnology Information (NCBI). These databases include nucleotide sequences, protein sequences, macromolecular structures, whole genomes, and MEDLINE through PubMed. Entrez provides access to the following databases:

- **PubMed:** Biomedical literature (PubMed),
  Web site: **http://www.ncbi.nlm.nih.gov/entrez/query.fcgi?db=PubMed**

- **Nucleotide Sequence Database (Genbank):**
  Web site:
  http://www.ncbi.nlm.nih.gov/entrez/query.fcgi?db=Nucleotide

- **Protein Sequence Database:**
  Web site: **http://www.ncbi.nlm.nih.gov/entrez/query.fcgi?db=Protein**

- **Structure:** Three-dimensional macromolecular structures,
  Web site: **http://www.ncbi.nlm.nih.gov/entrez/query.fcgi?db=Structure**

- **Genome:** Complete genome assemblies,
  Web site: **http://www.ncbi.nlm.nih.gov/entrez/query.fcgi?db=Genome**

- **PopSet:** Population study data sets,
  Web site: **http://www.ncbi.nlm.nih.gov/entrez/query.fcgi?db=Popset**

- **OMIM:** Online Mendelian Inheritance in Man,
  Web site: **http://www.ncbi.nlm.nih.gov/entrez/query.fcgi?db=OMIM**

- **Taxonomy:** Organisms in GenBank,
  Web site:
  http://www.ncbi.nlm.nih.gov/entrez/query.fcgi?db=Taxonomy

- **Books:** Online books,
  Web site: **http://www.ncbi.nlm.nih.gov/entrez/query.fcgi?db=books**

- **ProbeSet:** Gene Expression Omnibus (GEO),
  Web site: **http://www.ncbi.nlm.nih.gov/entrez/query.fcgi?db=geo**

- **3D Domains:** Domains from Entrez Structure,
  Web site: **http://www.ncbi.nlm.nih.gov/entrez/query.fcgi?db=geo**

- **NCBI's Protein Sequence Information Survey Results:**
  Web site: **http://www.ncbi.nlm.nih.gov/About/proteinsurvey/**

To access the Entrez system at the National Center for Biotechnology Information, go to **http://www.ncbi.nlm.nih.gov/entrez**, and then select the database that you would like to search. The databases available are listed in the drop box next to "Search." In the box next to "for," enter "immune thrombocytopenic purpura" (or synonyms) and click "Go."

Jablonski's Multiple Congenital Anomaly/Mental Retardation (MCA/MR) Syndromes Database[40]

This online resource can be quite useful. It has been developed to facilitate the identification and differentiation of syndromic entities. Special attention is given to the type of information that is usually limited or completely omitted in existing reference sources due to space limitations of the printed form.

At the following Web site you can also search synonyms alphabetically: **http://www.nlm.nih.gov/mesh/jablonski/syndrome_toc/toc_a.html.** You can search the MCA/MR database by keywords at this Web site: **http://www.nlm.nih.gov/mesh/jablonski/syndrome_db.html**.

The Genome Database[41]

Established at Johns Hopkins University in Baltimore, Maryland in 1990, the Genome Database (GDB) is the official central repository for genomic mapping data resulting from the Human Genome Initiative. In the spring of 1999, the Bioinformatics Supercomputing Centre (BiSC) at the Hospital for Sick Children in Toronto, Ontario assumed the management of GDB. The Human Genome Initiative is a worldwide research effort focusing on structural analysis of human DNA to determine the location and sequence of the estimated 100,000 human genes. In support of this project, GDB stores and curates data generated by researchers worldwide who are engaged in the mapping effort of the Human Genome Project (HGP). GDB's mission is to provide scientists with an encyclopedia of the human genome which is continually revised and updated to reflect the current state of scientific

---

[40] Adapted from the National Library of Medicine:
http://www.nlm.nih.gov/mesh/jablonski/about_syndrome.html.
[41] Adapted from the Genome Database:
http://gdbwww.gdb.org/gdb/aboutGDB.html#mission.

knowledge. Although GDB has historically focused on gene mapping, its focus will broaden as the Genome Project moves from mapping to sequence, and finally, to functional analysis.

To access the GDB, simply go to the following hyperlink: **http://www.gdb.org/**. Search "All Biological Data" by "Keyword." Type "immune thrombocytopenic purpura" (or synonyms) into the search box, and review the results. If more than one word is used in the search box, then separate each one with the word "and" or "or" (using "or" might be useful when using synonyms). This database is extremely technical as it was created for specialists. The articles are the results which are the most accessible to non-professionals and often listed under the heading "Citations." The contact names are also accessible to non-professionals.

Specialized References

The following books are specialized references written for professionals interested in immune thrombocytopenic purpura (sorted alphabetically by title, hyperlinks provide rankings, information, and reviews at Amazon.com):

- **Blood and Circulatory Disorders Sourcebook : Basic Information About Blood and Its Components (Health Reference Series, Vol 39)** by Linda M. Shin (Editor), Karen Bellenir (Editor); Library Binding - October 1998, Omnigraphics, Inc.; ISBN: 0780802039; **http://www.amazon.com/exec/obidos/ASIN/0780802039/icongroupinterna**

- **CRC Desk Reference for Hematology (CRC Desk Reference Series)** by N. K. Shinton (Editor); Hardcover - September 1998, CRC Press; ISBN: 0849396816; **http://www.amazon.com/exec/obidos/ASIN/0849396816/icongroupinterna**

- **Clinical Laboratory Hematology** by Shirlyn McKenzie; Hardcover - May 2002, Prentice Hall; ISBN: 0130199966; **http://www.amazon.com/exec/obidos/ASIN/0130199966/icongroupinterna**

- **Hematology for Students** by Archie A. MacKinney (Editor); (Paperback - June 2002), Harwood Academic Pub; ISBN: 9057026465; **http://www.amazon.com/exec/obidos/ASIN/9057026465/icongroupinterna**

- **Manual of Clinical Hematology** by Joseph J., MD Mazza (Editor); Spiral-bound, Lippincott, Williams & Wilkins Publishers; ISBN: 0781729807; **http://www.amazon.com/exec/obidos/ASIN/0781729807/icongroupinterna**

- **Microscopic Haematology: A Practical Guide for the Haematology Laboratory** by Gillian Rozenberg; Paperback - 160 pages (August 1, 1997),

Dunitz Martin Ltd.; ISBN: 9057022478;
http://www.amazon.com/exec/obidos/ASIN/9057022478/icongroupinterna

- **Pioneering Hematology : The Research & Treatment of Malignant Blood Disorders** by William C. Maloney; Hardcover - September 1997, Science History Publications; ISBN: 0881351954;
http://www.amazon.com/exec/obidos/ASIN/0881351954/icongroupinterna

- **Williams Hematology** by Ernest Beutler, M.D., Marshall A. Lichtman, M.D.; Hardcover - 1941 pages, 6th edition (November 28, 2000), McGraw-Hill Professional Publishing; ISBN: 0070703973;
http://www.amazon.com/exec/obidos/ASIN/0070703973/icongroupinterna

Vocabulary Builder

Adenosine: A nucleoside that is composed of adenine and d-ribose. Adenosine or adenosine derivatives play many important biological roles in addition to being components of DNA and RNA. Adenosine itself is a neurotransmitter. [NIH]

Malignant: Tending to become progressively worse and to result in death. Having the properties of anaplasia, invasion, and metastasis; said of tumours. [EU]

CHAPTER 9. DISSERTATIONS ON IMMUNE THROMBOCYTOPENIC PURPURA

Overview

University researchers are active in studying almost all known diseases. The result of research is often published in the form of Doctoral or Master's dissertations. You should understand, therefore, that applied diagnostic procedures and/or therapies can take many years to develop after the thesis that proposed the new technique or approach was written.

In this chapter, we will give you a bibliography on recent dissertations relating to immune thrombocytopenic purpura. You can read about these in more detail using the Internet or your local medical library. We will also provide you with information on how to use the Internet to stay current on dissertations.

Dissertations on Immune Thrombocytopenic Purpura

ProQuest Digital Dissertations is the largest archive of academic dissertations available. From this archive, we have compiled the following list covering dissertations devoted to immune thrombocytopenic purpura. You will see that the information provided includes the dissertation's title, its author, and the author's institution. To read more about the following, simply use the Internet address indicated. The following covers recent dissertations dealing with immune thrombocytopenic purpura:

- **Mechanisms Leading to Megakaryocyte Differentiation and Platelet Fragmentation** by Kaluzhny, Yulia; Phd from Boston University, 2002, 229 pages
  http://wwwlib.umi.com/dissertations/fullcit/3031578

- **The Expectations for the Future of Children with Hematologic Disorders and Their Mothers (sickle Cell Anemia, Itp)** by Schiller, Marilyn, Phd from New York University, 1989, 182 pages
  http://wwwlib.umi.com/dissertations/fullcit/9004322

Keeping Current

As previously mentioned, an effective way to stay current on dissertations dedicated to immune thrombocytopenic purpura is to use the database called *ProQuest Digital Dissertations* via the Internet, located at the following Web address: **http://wwwlib.umi.com/dissertations.** The site allows you to freely access the last two years of citations and abstracts. Ask your medical librarian if the library has full and unlimited access to this database. From the library, you should be able to do more complete searches than with the limited 2-year access available to the general public.

PART III. APPENDICES

ABOUT PART III

Part III is a collection of appendices on general medical topics which may be of interest to patients with immune thrombocytopenic purpura and related conditions.

APPENDIX A. RESEARCHING YOUR MEDICATIONS

Overview

There are a number of sources available on new or existing medications which could be prescribed to patients with immune thrombocytopenic purpura. While a number of hard copy or CD-Rom resources are available to patients and physicians for research purposes, a more flexible method is to use Internet-based databases. In this chapter, we will begin with a general overview of medications. We will then proceed to outline official recommendations on how you should view your medications. You may also want to research medications that you are currently taking for other conditions as they may interact with medications for immune thrombocytopenic purpura. Research can give you information on the side effects, interactions, and limitations of prescription drugs used in the treatment of immune thrombocytopenic purpura. Broadly speaking, there are two sources of information on approved medications: public sources and private sources. We will emphasize free-to-use public sources.

Your Medications: The Basics[42]

The Agency for Health Care Research and Quality has published extremely useful guidelines on how you can best participate in the medication aspects of immune thrombocytopenic purpura. Taking medicines is not always as simple as swallowing a pill. It can involve many steps and decisions each day. The AHCRQ recommends that patients with immune thrombocytopenic purpura take part in treatment decisions. Do not be afraid to ask questions and talk about your concerns. By taking a moment to ask questions early, you may avoid problems later. Here are some points to cover each time a new medicine is prescribed:

- Ask about all parts of your treatment, including diet changes, exercise, and medicines.

- Ask about the risks and benefits of each medicine or other treatment you might receive.

- Ask how often you or your doctor will check for side effects from a given medication.

Do not hesitate to ask what is important to you about your medicines. You may want a medicine with the fewest side effects, or the fewest doses to take each day. You may care most about cost, or how the medicine might affect how you live or work. Or, you may want the medicine your doctor believes will work the best. Telling your doctor will help him or her select the best treatment for you.

Do not be afraid to "bother" your doctor with your concerns and questions about medications for immune thrombocytopenic purpura. You can also talk to a nurse or a pharmacist. They can help you better understand your treatment plan. Feel free to bring a friend or family member with you when you visit your doctor. Talking over your options with someone you trust can help you make better choices, especially if you are not feeling well. Specifically, ask your doctor the following:

- The name of the medicine and what it is supposed to do.

- How and when to take the medicine, how much to take, and for how long.

- What food, drinks, other medicines, or activities you should avoid while taking the medicine.

- What side effects the medicine may have, and what to do if they occur.

---

[42] This section is adapted from AHCRQ: **http://www.ahcpr.gov/consumer/ncpiebro.htm**.

- If you can get a refill, and how often.

- About any terms or directions you do not understand.

- What to do if you miss a dose.

- If there is written information you can take home (most pharmacies have information sheets on your prescription medicines; some even offer large-print or Spanish versions).

Do not forget to tell your doctor about all the medicines you are currently taking (not just those for immune thrombocytopenic purpura). This includes prescription medicines and the medicines that you buy over the counter. Then your doctor can avoid giving you a new medicine that may not work well with the medications you take now. When talking to your doctor, you may wish to prepare a list of medicines you currently take, the reason you take them, and how you take them. Be sure to include the following information for each:

- Name of medicine

- Reason taken

- Dosage

- Time(s) of day

Also include any over-the-counter medicines, such as:

- Laxatives

- Diet pills

- Vitamins

- Cold medicine

- Aspirin or other pain, headache, or fever medicine

- Cough medicine

- Allergy relief medicine

- Antacids

- Sleeping pills

- Others (include names)

Learning More about Your Medications

Because of historical investments by various organizations and the emergence of the Internet, it has become rather simple to learn about the medications your doctor has recommended for immune thrombocytopenic purpura. One such source is the United States Pharmacopeia. In 1820, eleven physicians met in Washington, D.C. to establish the first compendium of standard drugs for the United States. They called this compendium the "U.S. Pharmacopeia (USP)." Today, the USP is a non-profit organization consisting of 800 volunteer scientists, eleven elected officials, and 400 representatives of state associations and colleges of medicine and pharmacy. The USP is located in Rockville, Maryland, and its home page is located at **www.usp.org**. The USP currently provides standards for over 3,700 medications. The resulting USP DI® Advice for the Patient® can be accessed through the National Library of Medicine of the National Institutes of Health. The database is partially derived from lists of federally approved medications in the Food and Drug Administration's (FDA) Drug Approvals database.[43]

While the FDA database is rather large and difficult to navigate, the Phamacopeia is both user-friendly and free to use. It covers more than 9,000 prescription and over-the-counter medications. To access this database, simply type the following hyperlink into your Web browser: **http://www.nlm.nih.gov/medlineplus/druginformation.html**. To view examples of a given medication (brand names, category, description, preparation, proper use, precautions, side effects, etc.), simply follow the hyperlinks indicated within the United States Pharmacopoeia. It is important to read the disclaimer by the United States Pharmacopoeia (**http://www.nlm.nih.gov/medlineplus/drugdisclaimer.html**) before using the information provided.

Of course, we as editors cannot be certain as to what medications you are taking. Therefore, we have compiled a list of medications associated with the treatment of immune thrombocytopenic purpura. Once again, due to space limitations, we only list a sample of medications and provide hyperlinks to ample documentation (e.g. typical dosage, side effects, drug-interaction risks, etc.). The following drugs have been mentioned in the Pharmacopeia and other sources as being potentially applicable to immune thrombocytopenic purpura:

---

[43] Though cumbersome, the FDA database can be freely browsed at the following site: **www.fda.gov/cder/da/da.htm**.

Rh O (D) Immune Globulin

- **Systemic - U.S. Brands:** MICRhoGAM; RhoGAM
  http://www.nlm.nih.gov/medlineplus/druginfo/rhodimmuneglo
  bulinsystemic202720.html

Commercial Databases

In addition to the medications listed in the USP above, a number of commercial sites are available by subscription to physicians and their institutions. You may be able to access these sources from your local medical library or your doctor's office.

Reuters Health Drug Database

The Reuters Health Drug Database can be searched by keyword at the hyperlink: **http://www.reutershealth.com/frame2/drug.html**. The following medications are listed in the Reuters' database as associated with immune thrombocytopenic purpura (including those with contraindications):[44]

- **Betamethasone**
  http://www.reutershealth.com/atoz/html/Betamethasone.htm

- **Corticotropin**
  http://www.reutershealth.com/atoz/html/Corticotropin.htm

- **Corticotropin (Adrenocorticotropic hormone; ACTH)**
  http://www.reutershealth.com/atoz/html/Corticotropin_(Adrenocortic
  otropic_hormone;_ACTH).htm

- **Dexamethasone**
  http://www.reutershealth.com/atoz/html/Dexamethasone.htm

- **Hydrocortisone (Cortisol)**
  http://www.reutershealth.com/atoz/html/Hydrocortisone_(Cortisol).htm

- **Immune Globulin Intravenous**
  http://www.reutershealth.com/atoz/html/Immune_Globulin_Intraven
  ous.htm

- **Immune Globulin Intravenous (IGIV)**
  http://www.reutershealth.com/atoz/html/Immune_Globulin_Intraven
  ous_(IGIV).htm

---

[44] Adapted from *A to Z Drug Facts* by Facts and Comparisons.

- **Immune Globulin IV**
  http://www.reutershealth.com/atoz/html/Immune_Globulin_IV.htm

- **Methylprednisolone**
  http://www.reutershealth.com/atoz/html/Methylprednisolone.htm

- **Pneumococcal Vaccine Polyvalent**
  http://www.reutershealth.com/atoz/html/Pneumococcal_Vaccine_Poly valent.htm

- **Prednisolone**
  http://www.reutershealth.com/atoz/html/Prednisolone.htm

- **Triamcinolone**
  http://www.reutershealth.com/atoz/html/Triamcinolone.htm

Mosby's GenRx

Mosby's GenRx database (also available on CD-Rom and book format) covers 45,000 drug products including generics and international brands. It provides prescribing information, drug interactions, and patient information. Information from the Mosby's GenRx database can be obtained at the following hyperlink: **http://www.genrx.com/Mosby/PhyGenRx/group.html**.

Physicians Desk Reference

The Physicians Desk Reference database (also available in CD-Rom and book format) is a full-text drug database. The database is searchable by brand name, generic name or by indication. It features multiple drug interactions reports. Information can be obtained at the following hyperlink: **http://physician.pdr.net/physician/templates/en/acl/psuser_t.htm**.

Other Web Sites

A number of additional Web sites discuss drug information. As an example, you may like to look at **www.drugs.com** which reproduces the information in the Pharmacopeia as well as commercial information. You may also want to consider the Web site of the Medical Letter, Inc. which allows users to download articles on various drugs and therapeutics for a nominal fee: **http://www.medletter.com/**.

Contraindications and Interactions (Hidden Dangers)

Some of the medications mentioned in the previous discussions can be problematic for patients with immune thrombocytopenic purpura--not because they are used in the treatment process, but because of contraindications, or side effects. Medications with contraindications are those that could react with drugs used to treat immune thrombocytopenic purpura or potentially create deleterious side effects in patients with immune thrombocytopenic purpura. You should ask your physician about any contraindications, especially as these might apply to other medications that you may be taking for common ailments.

Drug-drug interactions occur when two or more drugs react with each other. This drug-drug interaction may cause you to experience an unexpected side effect. Drug interactions may make your medications less effective, cause unexpected side effects, or increase the action of a particular drug. Some drug interactions can even be harmful to you.

Be sure to read the label every time you use a nonprescription or prescription drug, and take the time to learn about drug interactions. These precautions may be critical to your health. You can reduce the risk of potentially harmful drug interactions and side effects with a little bit of knowledge and common sense.

Drug labels contain important information about ingredients, uses, warnings, and directions which you should take the time to read and understand. Labels also include warnings about possible drug interactions. Further, drug labels may change as new information becomes available. This is why it's especially important to read the label every time you use a medication. When your doctor prescribes a new drug, discuss all over-the-counter and prescription medications, dietary supplements, vitamins, botanicals, minerals and herbals you take as well as the foods you eat. Ask your pharmacist for the package insert for each prescription drug you take. The package insert provides more information about potential drug interactions.

A Final Warning

At some point, you may hear of alternative medications from friends, relatives, or in the news media. Advertisements may suggest that certain alternative drugs can produce positive results for patients with immune thrombocytopenic purpura. Exercise caution--some of these drugs may have fraudulent claims, and others may actually hurt you. The Food and Drug Administration (FDA) is the official U.S. agency charged with discovering which medications are likely to improve the health of patients with immune thrombocytopenic purpura. The FDA warns patients to watch out for[45]:

- Secret formulas (real scientists share what they know)

- Amazing breakthroughs or miracle cures (real breakthroughs don't happen very often; when they do, real scientists do not call them amazing or miracles)

- Quick, painless, or guaranteed cures

- If it sounds too good to be true, it probably isn't true.

If you have any questions about any kind of medical treatment, the FDA may have an office near you. Look for their number in the blue pages of the phone book. You can also contact the FDA through its toll-free number, 1-888-INFO-FDA (1-888-463-6332), or on the World Wide Web at **www.fda.gov**.

General References

In addition to the resources provided earlier in this chapter, the following general references describe medications (sorted alphabetically by title; hyperlinks provide rankings, information and reviews at Amazon.com):

- **Complete Guide to Prescription and Nonprescription Drugs 2001 (Complete Guide to Prescription and Nonprescription Drugs, 2001)** by H. Winter Griffith, Paperback 16th edition (2001), Medical Surveillance; ISBN: 0942447417;
  http://www.amazon.com/exec/obidos/ASIN/039952634X/icongroupinterna

- **The Essential Guide to Prescription Drugs, 2001** by James J. Rybacki, James W. Long; Paperback - 1274 pages (2001), Harper Resource; ISBN: 0060958162;
  http://www.amazon.com/exec/obidos/ASIN/0060958162/icongroupinterna

- **Handbook of Commonly Prescribed Drugs** by G. John Digregorio, Edward J. Barbieri; Paperback 16th edition (2001), Medical Surveillance; ISBN: 0942447417;
  http://www.amazon.com/exec/obidos/ASIN/0942447417/icongroupinterna

---

[45] This section has been adapted from http://www.fda.gov/opacom/lowlit/medfraud.html.

- **Johns Hopkins Complete Home Encyclopedia of Drugs 2nd ed.** by Simeon Margolis (Ed.), Johns Hopkins; Hardcover - 835 pages (2000), Rebus; ISBN: 0929661583;
  http://www.amazon.com/exec/obidos/ASIN/0929661583/icongroupinterna

- **Medical Pocket Reference: Drugs 2002** by Springhouse Paperback 1st edition (2001), Lippincott Williams & Wilkins Publishers; ISBN: 1582550964;
  http://www.amazon.com/exec/obidos/ASIN/1582550964/icongroupinterna

- **PDR** by Medical Economics Staff, Medical Economics Staff Hardcover - 3506 pages 55th edition (2000), Medical Economics Company; ISBN: 1563633752;
  http://www.amazon.com/exec/obidos/ASIN/1563633752/icongroupinterna

- **Pharmacy Simplified: A Glossary of Terms** by James Grogan; Paperback - 432 pages, 1st edition (2001), Delmar Publishers; ISBN: 0766828581;
  http://www.amazon.com/exec/obidos/ASIN/0766828581/icongroupinterna

- **Physician Federal Desk Reference** by Christine B. Fraizer; Paperback 2nd edition (2001), Medicode Inc; ISBN: 1563373971;
  http://www.amazon.com/exec/obidos/ASIN/1563373971/icongroupinterna

- **Physician's Desk Reference Supplements** Paperback - 300 pages, 53 edition (1999), ISBN: 1563632950;
  http://www.amazon.com/exec/obidos/ASIN/1563632950/icongroupinterna

APPENDIX B. RESEARCHING ALTERNATIVE MEDICINE

Overview

Complementary and alternative medicine (CAM) is one of the most contentious aspects of modern medical practice. You may have heard of these treatments on the radio or on television. Maybe you have seen articles written about these treatments in magazines, newspapers, or books. Perhaps your friends or doctor have mentioned alternatives.

In this chapter, we will begin by giving you a broad perspective on complementary and alternative therapies. Next, we will introduce you to official information sources on CAM relating to immune thrombocytopenic purpura. Finally, at the conclusion of this chapter, we will provide a list of readings on immune thrombocytopenic purpura from various authors. We will begin, however, with the National Center for Complementary and Alternative Medicine's (NCCAM) overview of complementary and alternative medicine.

What Is CAM?[46]

Complementary and alternative medicine (CAM) covers a broad range of healing philosophies, approaches, and therapies. Generally, it is defined as those treatments and healthcare practices which are not taught in medical schools, used in hospitals, or reimbursed by medical insurance companies. Many CAM therapies are termed "holistic," which generally means that the healthcare practitioner considers the whole person, including physical, mental, emotional, and spiritual health. Some of these therapies are also

---

[46] Adapted from the NCCAM: **http://nccam.nih.gov/nccam/fcp/faq/index.html#what-is**.

known as "preventive," which means that the practitioner educates and treats the person to prevent health problems from arising, rather than treating symptoms after problems have occurred.

People use CAM treatments and therapies in a variety of ways. Therapies are used alone (often referred to as alternative), in combination with other alternative therapies, or in addition to conventional treatment (sometimes referred to as complementary). Complementary and alternative medicine, or "integrative medicine," includes a broad range of healing philosophies, approaches, and therapies. Some approaches are consistent with physiological principles of Western medicine, while others constitute healing systems with non-Western origins. While some therapies are far outside the realm of accepted Western medical theory and practice, others are becoming established in mainstream medicine.

Complementary and alternative therapies are used in an effort to prevent illness, reduce stress, prevent or reduce side effects and symptoms, or control or cure disease. Some commonly used methods of complementary or alternative therapy include mind/body control interventions such as visualization and relaxation, manual healing including acupressure and massage, homeopathy, vitamins or herbal products, and acupuncture.

What Are the Domains of Alternative Medicine?[47]

The list of CAM practices changes continually. The reason being is that these new practices and therapies are often proved to be safe and effective, and therefore become generally accepted as "mainstream" healthcare practices. Today, CAM practices may be grouped within five major domains: (1) alternative medical systems, (2) mind-body interventions, (3) biologically-based treatments, (4) manipulative and body-based methods, and (5) energy therapies. The individual systems and treatments comprising these categories are too numerous to list in this sourcebook. Thus, only limited examples are provided within each.

Alternative Medical Systems

Alternative medical systems involve complete systems of theory and practice that have evolved independent of, and often prior to, conventional biomedical approaches. Many are traditional systems of medicine that are

---

[47] Adapted from the NCCAM: http://nccam.nih.gov/nccam/fcp/classify/index.html.

practiced by individual cultures throughout the world, including a number of venerable Asian approaches.

Traditional oriental medicine emphasizes the balance or disturbances of qi (pronounced chi) or vital energy in health and disease, respectively. Traditional oriental medicine consists of a group of techniques and methods including acupuncture, herbal medicine, oriental massage, and qi gong (a form of energy therapy). Acupuncture involves stimulating specific anatomic points in the body for therapeutic purposes, usually by puncturing the skin with a thin needle.

Ayurveda is India's traditional system of medicine. Ayurvedic medicine (meaning "science of life") is a comprehensive system of medicine that places equal emphasis on body, mind, and spirit. Ayurveda strives to restore the innate harmony of the individual. Some of the primary Ayurvedic treatments include diet, exercise, meditation, herbs, massage, exposure to sunlight, and controlled breathing.

Other traditional healing systems have been developed by the world's indigenous populations. These populations include Native American, Aboriginal, African, Middle Eastern, Tibetan, and Central and South American cultures. Homeopathy and naturopathy are also examples of complete alternative medicine systems.

Homeopathic medicine is an unconventional Western system that is based on the principle that "like cures like," i.e., that the same substance that in large doses produces the symptoms of an illness, in very minute doses cures it. Homeopathic health practitioners believe that the more dilute the remedy, the greater its potency. Therefore, they use small doses of specially prepared plant extracts and minerals to stimulate the body's defense mechanisms and healing processes in order to treat illness.

Naturopathic medicine is based on the theory that disease is a manifestation of alterations in the processes by which the body naturally heals itself and emphasizes health restoration rather than disease treatment. Naturopathic physicians employ an array of healing practices, including the following: diet and clinical nutrition, homeopathy, acupuncture, herbal medicine, hydrotherapy (the use of water in a range of temperatures and methods of applications), spinal and soft-tissue manipulation, physical therapies (such as those involving electrical currents, ultrasound, and light), therapeutic counseling, and pharmacology.

Mind-Body Interventions

Mind-body interventions employ a variety of techniques designed to facilitate the mind's capacity to affect bodily function and symptoms. Only a select group of mind-body interventions having well-documented theoretical foundations are considered CAM. For example, patient education and cognitive-behavioral approaches are now considered "mainstream." On the other hand, complementary and alternative medicine includes meditation, certain uses of hypnosis, dance, music, and art therapy, as well as prayer and mental healing.

Biological-Based Therapies

This category of CAM includes natural and biological-based practices, interventions, and products, many of which overlap with conventional medicine's use of dietary supplements. This category includes herbal, special dietary, orthomolecular, and individual biological therapies.

Herbal therapy employs an individual herb or a mixture of herbs for healing purposes. An herb is a plant or plant part that produces and contains chemical substances that act upon the body. Special diet therapies, such as those proposed by Drs. Atkins, Ornish, Pritikin, and Weil, are believed to prevent and/or control illness as well as promote health. Orthomolecular therapies aim to treat disease with varying concentrations of chemicals such as magnesium, melatonin, and mega-doses of vitamins. Biological therapies include, for example, the use of laetrile and shark cartilage to treat cancer and the use of bee pollen to treat autoimmune and inflammatory diseases.

Manipulative and Body-Based Methods

This category includes methods that are based on manipulation and/or movement of the body. For example, chiropractors focus on the relationship between structure and function, primarily pertaining to the spine, and how that relationship affects the preservation and restoration of health. Chiropractors use manipulative therapy as an integral treatment tool.

In contrast, osteopaths place particular emphasis on the musculoskeletal system and practice osteopathic manipulation. Osteopaths believe that all of the body's systems work together and that disturbances in one system may have an impact upon function elsewhere in the body. Massage therapists manipulate the soft tissues of the body to normalize those tissues.

Energy Therapies

Energy therapies focus on energy fields originating within the body (biofields) or those from other sources (electromagnetic fields). Biofield therapies are intended to affect energy fields (the existence of which is not yet experimentally proven) that surround and penetrate the human body. Some forms of energy therapy manipulate biofields by applying pressure and/or manipulating the body by placing the hands in or through these fields. Examples include Qi gong, Reiki and Therapeutic Touch.

Qi gong is a component of traditional oriental medicine that combines movement, meditation, and regulation of breathing to enhance the flow of vital energy (qi) in the body, improve blood circulation, and enhance immune function. Reiki, the Japanese word representing Universal Life Energy, is based on the belief that, by channeling spiritual energy through the practitioner, the spirit is healed and, in turn, heals the physical body. Therapeutic Touch is derived from the ancient technique of "laying-on of hands." It is based on the premises that the therapist's healing force affects the patient's recovery and that healing is promoted when the body's energies are in balance. By passing their hands over the patient, these healers identify energy imbalances.

Bioelectromagnetic-based therapies involve the unconventional use of electromagnetic fields to treat illnesses or manage pain. These therapies are often used to treat asthma, cancer, and migraine headaches. Types of electromagnetic fields which are manipulated in these therapies include pulsed fields, magnetic fields, and alternating current or direct current fields.

Can Alternatives Affect My Treatment?

A critical issue in pursuing complementary alternatives mentioned thus far is the risk that these might have undesirable interactions with your medical treatment. It becomes all the more important to speak with your doctor who can offer advice on the use of alternatives. Official sources confirm this view. Though written for women, we find that the National Women's Health Information Center's advice on pursuing alternative medicine is appropriate for patients of both genders and all ages.[48]

---

[48] Adapted from **http://www.4woman.gov/faq/alternative.htm**.

Is It Okay to Want Both Traditional and Alternative Medicine?

Should you wish to explore non-traditional types of treatment, be sure to discuss all issues concerning treatments and therapies with your healthcare provider, whether a physician or practitioner of complementary and alternative medicine. Competent healthcare management requires knowledge of both conventional and alternative therapies you are taking for the practitioner to have a complete picture of your treatment plan.

The decision to use complementary and alternative treatments is an important one. Consider before selecting an alternative therapy, the safety and effectiveness of the therapy or treatment, the expertise and qualifications of the healthcare practitioner, and the quality of delivery. These topics should be considered when selecting any practitioner or therapy.

Finding CAM References on Immune Thrombocytopenic Purpura

Having read the previous discussion, you may be wondering which complementary or alternative treatments might be appropriate for immune thrombocytopenic purpura. For the remainder of this chapter, we will direct you to a number of official sources which can assist you in researching studies and publications. Some of these articles are rather technical, so some patience may be required.

National Center for Complementary and Alternative Medicine

The National Center for Complementary and Alternative Medicine (NCCAM) of the National Institutes of Health (**http://nccam.nih.gov**) has created a link to the National Library of Medicine's databases to allow patients to search for articles that specifically relate to immune thrombocytopenic purpura and complementary medicine. To search the database, go to **www.nlm.nih.gov/nccam/camonpubmed.html**. Select "CAM on PubMed." Enter "immune thrombocytopenic purpura" (or synonyms) into the search box. Click "Go." The following references provide information on particular aspects of complementary and alternative medicine (CAM) that are related to immune thrombocytopenic purpura:

- **A human monoclonal autoantibody specific for human platelet glycoprotein IIb (integrin alpha IIb) heavy chain.**
  Author(s): Kunicki TJ, Furihata K, Kekomaki R, Scott JP, Nugent DJ.

Source: Hum Antibodies Hybridomas. 1990; 1(2): 83-95.
http://www.ncbi.nlm.nih.gov:80/entrez/query.fcgi?cmd=Retrieve&db=PubMed&list_uids=1715776&dopt=Abstract

- **Allogeneic stem cell transplantation for Evans syndrome.**
  Author(s): Oyama Y, Papadopoulos EB, Miranda M, Traynor AE, Burt RK.
  Source: Bone Marrow Transplantation. 2001 November; 28(9): 903-5. Review.
  http://www.ncbi.nlm.nih.gov:80/entrez/query.fcgi?cmd=Retrieve&db=PubMed&list_uids=11781654&dopt=Abstract

- **Cascade filtration for TTP: an effective alternative to plasma exchange with cryodepleted plasma.**
  Author(s): Bruni R, Giannini G, Lercari G, Bo A, Florio G, De Luigi MC, Marmont A, Gobbi A, Damasio E, Valbonesi M.
  Source: Transfusion Science. 1999 December; 21(3): 193-9.
  http://www.ncbi.nlm.nih.gov:80/entrez/query.fcgi?cmd=Retrieve&db=PubMed&list_uids=10848440&dopt=Abstract

- **Combination chemotherapy in refractory immune thrombocytopenic purpura.**
  Author(s): Figueroa M, Gehlsen J, Hammond D, Ondreyco S, Piro L, Pomeroy T, Williams F, McMillan R.
  Source: The New England Journal of Medicine. 1993 April 29; 328(17): 1226-9.
  http://www.ncbi.nlm.nih.gov:80/entrez/query.fcgi?cmd=Retrieve&db=PubMed&list_uids=8464433&dopt=Abstract

- **Durable response to etoposide-loaded platelets in refractory immune thrombocytopenic purpura: a case report.**
  Author(s): Wood L, Jacobs P.
  Source: American Journal of Hematology. 1988 January; 27(1): 63-4.
  http://www.ncbi.nlm.nih.gov:80/entrez/query.fcgi?cmd=Retrieve&db=PubMed&list_uids=3354557&dopt=Abstract

- **Effect of danazol in immune thrombocytopenic purpura.**
  Author(s): Schreiber AD, Chien P, Tomaski A, Cines DB.

Source: The New England Journal of Medicine. 1987 February 26; 316(9): 503-8.
http://www.ncbi.nlm.nih.gov:80/entrez/query.fcgi?cmd=Retrieve&db=PubMed&list_uids=3807993&dopt=Abstract

- **Effects of kami-kihi-to (jia-wei-gui-pi-tang) on autoantibodies in patients with chronic immune thrombocytopenic purpura.**
  Author(s): Yamaguchi K, Kido H, Kawakatsu T, Fukuroi T, Suzuki M, Yanabu M, Nomura S, Kokawa T, Yasunaga K.
  Source: Am J Chin Med. 1993; 21(3-4): 251-5.
  http://www.ncbi.nlm.nih.gov:80/entrez/query.fcgi?cmd=Retrieve&db=PubMed&list_uids=8135169&dopt=Abstract

- **Glycocalicin: a new assay--the normal plasma levels and its potential usefulness in selected diseases.**
  Author(s): Beer JH, Buchi L, Steiner B.
  Source: Blood. 1994 February 1; 83(3): 691-702.
  http://www.ncbi.nlm.nih.gov:80/entrez/query.fcgi?cmd=Retrieve&db=PubMed&list_uids=8298132&dopt=Abstract

- **Immune thrombocytopenia after umbilical cord progenitor cell transplant: response to vincristine.**
  Author(s): Dovat S, Roberts RL, Wakim M, Stiehm ER, Feig SA.
  Source: Bone Marrow Transplantation. 1999 August; 24(3): 321-3.
  http://www.ncbi.nlm.nih.gov:80/entrez/query.fcgi?cmd=Retrieve&db=PubMed&list_uids=10455373&dopt=Abstract

- **Immune thrombocytopenia and hemolytic anemia as a presenting manifestation of Hodgkin disease.**
  Author(s): Ertem M, Uysal Z, Yavuz G, Gozdasoglu S.
  Source: Pediatric Hematology and Oncology. 2000 March; 17(2): 181-5.
  http://www.ncbi.nlm.nih.gov:80/entrez/query.fcgi?cmd=Retrieve&db=PubMed&list_uids=10734662&dopt=Abstract

- **Immunologic and clinical investigation on a bovine thymic extract. Therapeutic applications in primary immunoedificiencies.**
  Author(s): Aiuti F, Ammirati P, Fiorilli M, D'Amelio R, Franchi F, Calvani M, Businco L.
  Source: Pediatric Research. 1979 July; 13(7): 797-802.
  http://www.ncbi.nlm.nih.gov:80/entrez/query.fcgi?cmd=Retrieve&db=PubMed&list_uids=314621&dopt=Abstract

- **Immunosuppressive therapy of idiopathic thrombocytopenic purpura.**
  Author(s): Caplan SN, Berkman EM.
  Source: The Medical Clinics of North America. 1976 September; 60(5): 971-86. Review.
  http://www.ncbi.nlm.nih.gov:80/entrez/query.fcgi?cmd=Retrieve&db= PubMed&list_uids=781417&dopt=Abstract

- **Initial management of immune thrombocytopenic purpura in children: is supportive counseling without therapeutic intervention sufficient?**
  Author(s): George JN.
  Source: The Journal of Pediatrics. 2000 November; 137(5): 598-600. No Abstract Available.
  http://www.ncbi.nlm.nih.gov:80/entrez/query.fcgi?cmd=Retrieve&db= PubMed&list_uids=11060520&dopt=Abstract

- **Management of auricular hematoma using a thermoplastic splint.**
  Author(s): Henderson JM, Salama AR, Blanchaert RH Jr.
  Source: Archives of Otolaryngology--Head & Neck Surgery. 2000 July; 126(7): 888-90.
  http://www.ncbi.nlm.nih.gov:80/entrez/query.fcgi?cmd=Retrieve&db= PubMed&list_uids=10889002&dopt=Abstract

- **Overview of idiopathic thrombocytopenic purpura: new approach to refractory patients.**
  Author(s): Bussel JB.
  Source: Seminars in Oncology. 2000 December; 27(6 Suppl 12): 91-8. Review.
  http://www.ncbi.nlm.nih.gov:80/entrez/query.fcgi?cmd=Retrieve&db= PubMed&list_uids=11226007&dopt=Abstract

- **Platelet autoantibodies in immune thrombocytopenic purpura.**
  Author(s): Beardsley DS, Ertem M.
  Source: Transfusion Science. 1998 September; 19(3): 237-44. Review.
  http://www.ncbi.nlm.nih.gov:80/entrez/query.fcgi?cmd=Retrieve&db= PubMed&list_uids=10351135&dopt=Abstract

- **Platelet-associated antibody to glycoprotein IIb/IIIa from chronic immune thrombocytopenic purpura patients often binds to divalent cation-dependent antigens.**
  Author(s): Fujisawa K, Tani P, McMillan R.

Source: Blood. 1993 March 1; 81(5): 1284-9.
http://www.ncbi.nlm.nih.gov:80/entrez/query.fcgi?cmd=Retrieve&db=
PubMed&list_uids=7680243&dopt=Abstract

- **Platelet-associated anti-glycoprotein (GP) IIb-IIIa autoantibodies in chronic immune thrombocytopenic purpura mainly recognize cation-dependent conformations: comparison with the epitopes of serum autoantibodies.**
  Author(s): Kosugi S, Tomiyama Y, Shiraga M, Kashiwagi H, Mizutani H, Kanakura Y, Kurata Y, Matsuzawa Y.
  Source: Thrombosis and Haemostasis. 1996 February; 75(2): 339-45.
  http://www.ncbi.nlm.nih.gov:80/entrez/query.fcgi?cmd=Retrieve&db=
  PubMed&list_uids=8815587&dopt=Abstract

- **Quantitation of platelet-associated IgG by radial immunodiffusion.**
  Author(s): Morse BS, Giuliani D, Nussbaum M.
  Source: Blood. 1981 April; 57(4): 809-11.
  http://www.ncbi.nlm.nih.gov:80/entrez/query.fcgi?cmd=Retrieve&db=
  PubMed&list_uids=6781555&dopt=Abstract

- **Reactivity of autoantibodies from chronic ITP patients with recombinant glycoprotein IIIa peptides.**
  Author(s): Bowditch RD, Tani P, McMillan R.
  Source: British Journal of Haematology. 1995 September; 91(1): 178-84.
  http://www.ncbi.nlm.nih.gov:80/entrez/query.fcgi?cmd=Retrieve&db=
  PubMed&list_uids=7577629&dopt=Abstract

- **Reticulated platelet counts in the diagnosis of acute immune thrombocytopenic purpura.**
  Author(s): Saxon BR, Blanchette VS, Butchart S, Lim-Yin J, Poon AO.
  Source: Journal of Pediatric Hematology/Oncology : Official Journal of the American Society of Pediatric Hematology/Oncology. 1998 January-February; 20(1): 44-8.
  http://www.ncbi.nlm.nih.gov:80/entrez/query.fcgi?cmd=Retrieve&db=
  PubMed&list_uids=9482412&dopt=Abstract

- **Targeted-immunosuppression with vincristine infusion in the treatment of immune thrombocytopenia.**
  Author(s): Manoharan A.

Source: Aust N Z J Med. 1991 August; 21(4): 405-7.
http://www.ncbi.nlm.nih.gov:80/entrez/query.fcgi?cmd=Retrieve&db=PubMed&list_uids=1953528&dopt=Abstract

- **The effect of therapy on platelet-associated autoantibody in chronic immune thrombocytopenic purpura.**
  Author(s): Fujisawa K, Tani P, Piro L, McMillan R.
  Source: Blood. 1993 June 1; 81(11): 2872-7.
  http://www.ncbi.nlm.nih.gov:80/entrez/query.fcgi?cmd=Retrieve&db=PubMed&list_uids=8499625&dopt=Abstract

- **The use of vincristine in refractory auto-immune thrombocytopenic purpura.**
  Author(s): Van Zyl-Smit R, Jacobs P.
  Source: South African Medical Journal. Suid-Afrikaanse Tydskrif Vir Geneeskunde. 1974 October 5; 48(48): 2039-41. No Abstract Available.
  http://www.ncbi.nlm.nih.gov:80/entrez/query.fcgi?cmd=Retrieve&db=PubMed&list_uids=4474709&dopt=Abstract

- **Treatment of chronic immune thrombocytopenia.**
  Author(s): Rosse WF.
  Source: Clin Haematol. 1983 February; 12(1): 267-84. Review. No Abstract Available.
  http://www.ncbi.nlm.nih.gov:80/entrez/query.fcgi?cmd=Retrieve&db=PubMed&list_uids=6340883&dopt=Abstract

- **Vincristine by infusion for childhood acute immune thrombocytopenia.**
  Author(s): Manoharan A.
  Source: Lancet. 1986 February 8; 1(8476): 317. No Abstract Available.
  http://www.ncbi.nlm.nih.gov:80/entrez/query.fcgi?cmd=Retrieve&db=PubMed&list_uids=2868175&dopt=Abstract

- **Vincristine for childhood immune thrombocytopenia.**
  Author(s): Lilleyman JS.
  Source: Lancet. 1986 March 1; 1(8479): 499. No Abstract Available.
  http://www.ncbi.nlm.nih.gov:80/entrez/query.fcgi?cmd=Retrieve&db=PubMed&list_uids=2869232&dopt=Abstract

Additional Web Resources

A number of additional Web sites offer encyclopedic information covering CAM and related topics. The following is a representative sample:

- Alternative Medicine Foundation, Inc.: **http://www.herbmed.org/**

- AOL: **http://search.aol.com/cat.adp?id=169&layer=&from=subcats**

- Chinese Medicine: **http://www.newcenturynutrition.com/**

- drkoop.com®:
  http://www.drkoop.com/InteractiveMedicine/IndexC.html

- Family Village: **http://www.familyvillage.wisc.edu/med_altn.htm**

- Google: **http://directory.google.com/Top/Health/Alternative/**

- Healthnotes: **http://www.thedacare.org/healthnotes/**

- Open Directory Project: **http://dmoz.org/Health/Alternative/**

- TPN.com: **http://www.tnp.com/**

- Yahoo.com: **http://dir.yahoo.com/Health/Alternative_Medicine/**

- WebMD®Health: **http://my.webmd.com/drugs_and_herbs**

- WellNet: **http://www.wellnet.ca/herbsa-c.htm**

- WholeHealthMD.com:
  http://www.wholehealthmd.com/reflib/0,1529,,00.html

General References

A good place to find general background information on CAM is the National Library of Medicine. It has prepared within the MEDLINEplus system an information topic page dedicated to complementary and alternative medicine. To access this page, go to the MEDLINEplus site at: **http://www.nlm.nih.gov/medlineplus/alternativemedicine.html.** This Web site provides a general overview of various topics and can lead to a number of general sources. The following additional references describe, in broad terms, alternative and complementary medicine (sorted alphabetically by title; hyperlinks provide rankings, information, and reviews at Amazon.com):

- **Chelation Therapy and Your Health: This Noninvasive Treatment for Vascular Disease Reduces Free Radical Damage to Blood Vessels** by Michael Janson; Paperback - 48 pages (December 1998), McGraw Hill -

NTC; ISBN: 087983899X;
http://www.amazon.com/exec/obidos/ASIN/087983899X/icongroupinterna

- **Handbook of Chinese Hematology** by Simon Becker; Paperback - 250 pages (June 1, 2000), Blue Poppy Press; ISBN: 1891845160; http://www.amazon.com/exec/obidos/ASIN/1891845160/icongroupinterna

- **A Textbook on Edta Chelation Therapy** by Elmer M. Cranton (Editor), Linus Pauling; Hardcover - April 2001, Hampton Roads Pub Co; ISBN: 1571742530; http://www.amazon.com/exec/obidos/ASIN/1571742530/icongroupinterna

For additional information on complementary and alternative medicine, ask your doctor or write to:

National Institutes of Health
National Center for Complementary and Alternative Medicine Clearinghouse
P. O. Box 8218
Silver Spring, MD 20907-8218

Vocabulary Builder

The following vocabulary builder gives definitions of words used in this chapter that have not been defined in previous chapters:

Auricular: Pertaining to an auricle or to the ear, and, formerly, to an atrium of the heart. [EU]

Hematoma: An extravasation of blood localized in an organ, space, or tissue. [NIH]

Hybridomas: Cells artificially created by fusion of activated lymphocytes with neoplastic cells. The resulting hybrid cells are cloned and produce pure or "monoclonal" antibodies or T-cell products, identical to those produced by the immunologically competent parent, and continually grow and divide as the neoplastic parent. [NIH]

Immunodiffusion: Technique involving the diffusion of antigen or antibody through a semisolid medium, usually agar or agarose gel, with the result being a precipitin reaction. [NIH]

Otolaryngology: A surgical specialty concerned with the study and treatment of disorders of the ear, nose, and throat. [NIH]

APPENDIX C. RESEARCHING NUTRITION

Overview

Since the time of Hippocrates, doctors have understood the importance of diet and nutrition to patients' health and well-being. Since then, they have accumulated an impressive archive of studies and knowledge dedicated to this subject. Based on their experience, doctors and healthcare providers may recommend particular dietary supplements to patients with immune thrombocytopenic purpura. Any dietary recommendation is based on a patient's age, body mass, gender, lifestyle, eating habits, food preferences, and health condition. It is therefore likely that different patients with immune thrombocytopenic purpura may be given different recommendations. Some recommendations may be directly related to immune thrombocytopenic purpura, while others may be more related to the patient's general health. These recommendations, themselves, may differ from what official sources recommend for the average person.

In this chapter we will begin by briefly reviewing the essentials of diet and nutrition that will broadly frame more detailed discussions of immune thrombocytopenic purpura. We will then show you how to find studies dedicated specifically to nutrition and immune thrombocytopenic purpura.

Food and Nutrition: General Principles

What Are Essential Foods?

Food is generally viewed by official sources as consisting of six basic elements: (1) fluids, (2) carbohydrates, (3) protein, (4) fats, (5) vitamins, and

(6) minerals. Consuming a combination of these elements is considered to be a healthy diet:

- **Fluids** are essential to human life as 80-percent of the body is composed of water. Water is lost via urination, sweating, diarrhea, vomiting, diuretics (drugs that increase urination), caffeine, and physical exertion.

- **Carbohydrates** are the main source for human energy (thermoregulation) and the bulk of typical diets. They are mostly classified as being either simple or complex. Simple carbohydrates include sugars which are often consumed in the form of cookies, candies, or cakes. Complex carbohydrates consist of starches and dietary fibers. Starches are consumed in the form of pastas, breads, potatoes, rice, and other foods. Soluble fibers can be eaten in the form of certain vegetables, fruits, oats, and legumes. Insoluble fibers include brown rice, whole grains, certain fruits, wheat bran and legumes.

- **Proteins** are eaten to build and repair human tissues. Some foods that are high in protein are also high in fat and calories. Food sources for protein include nuts, meat, fish, cheese, and other dairy products.

- **Fats** are consumed for both energy and the absorption of certain vitamins. There are many types of fats, with many general publications recommending the intake of unsaturated fats or those low in cholesterol.

Vitamins and minerals are fundamental to human health, growth, and, in some cases, disease prevention. Most are consumed in your diet (exceptions being vitamins K and D which are produced by intestinal bacteria and sunlight on the skin, respectively). Each vitamin and mineral plays a different role in health. The following outlines essential vitamins:

- **Vitamin A** is important to the health of your eyes, hair, bones, and skin; sources of vitamin A include foods such as eggs, carrots, and cantaloupe.

- **Vitamin B^1**, also known as thiamine, is important for your nervous system and energy production; food sources for thiamine include meat, peas, fortified cereals, bread, and whole grains.

- **Vitamin B^2**, also known as riboflavin, is important for your nervous system and muscles, but is also involved in the release of proteins from nutrients; food sources for riboflavin include dairy products, leafy vegetables, meat, and eggs.

- **Vitamin B^3**, also known as niacin, is important for healthy skin and helps the body use energy; food sources for niacin include peas, peanuts, fish, and whole grains

- **Vitamin B^6**, also known as pyridoxine, is important for the regulation of cells in the nervous system and is vital for blood formation; food sources for pyridoxine include bananas, whole grains, meat, and fish.

- **Vitamin B^{12}** is vital for a healthy nervous system and for the growth of red blood cells in bone marrow; food sources for vitamin B^{12} include yeast, milk, fish, eggs, and meat.

- **Vitamin C** allows the body's immune system to fight various diseases, strengthens body tissue, and improves the body's use of iron; food sources for vitamin C include a wide variety of fruits and vegetables.

- **Vitamin D** helps the body absorb calcium which strengthens bones and teeth; food sources for vitamin D include oily fish and dairy products.

- **Vitamin E** can help protect certain organs and tissues from various degenerative diseases; food sources for vitamin E include margarine, vegetables, eggs, and fish.

- **Vitamin K** is essential for bone formation and blood clotting; common food sources for vitamin K include leafy green vegetables.

- **Folic Acid** maintains healthy cells and blood and, when taken by a pregnant woman, can prevent her fetus from developing neural tube defects; food sources for folic acid include nuts, fortified breads, leafy green vegetables, and whole grains.

It should be noted that one can overdose on certain vitamins which become toxic if consumed in excess (e.g. vitamin A, D, E and K).

Like vitamins, minerals are chemicals that are required by the body to remain in good health. Because the human body does not manufacture these chemicals internally, we obtain them from food and other dietary sources. The more important minerals include:

- **Calcium** is needed for healthy bones, teeth, and muscles, but also helps the nervous system function; food sources for calcium include dry beans, peas, eggs, and dairy products.

- **Chromium** is helpful in regulating sugar levels in blood; food sources for chromium include egg yolks, raw sugar, cheese, nuts, beets, whole grains, and meat.

- **Fluoride** is used by the body to help prevent tooth decay and to reinforce bone strength; sources of fluoride include drinking water and certain brands of toothpaste.

- **Iodine** helps regulate the body's use of energy by synthesizing into the hormone thyroxine; food sources include leafy green vegetables, nuts, egg yolks, and red meat.

- **Iron** helps maintain muscles and the formation of red blood cells and certain proteins; food sources for iron include meat, dairy products, eggs, and leafy green vegetables.

- **Magnesium** is important for the production of DNA, as well as for healthy teeth, bones, muscles, and nerves; food sources for magnesium include dried fruit, dark green vegetables, nuts, and seafood.

- **Phosphorous** is used by the body to work with calcium to form bones and teeth; food sources for phosphorous include eggs, meat, cereals, and dairy products.

- **Selenium** primarily helps maintain normal heart and liver functions; food sources for selenium include wholegrain cereals, fish, meat, and dairy products.

- **Zinc** helps wounds heal, the formation of sperm, and encourage rapid growth and energy; food sources include dried beans, shellfish, eggs, and nuts.

The United States government periodically publishes recommended diets and consumption levels of the various elements of food. Again, your doctor may encourage deviations from the average official recommendation based on your specific condition. To learn more about basic dietary guidelines, visit the Web site: **http://www.health.gov/dietaryguidelines/**. Based on these guidelines, many foods are required to list the nutrition levels on the food's packaging. Labeling Requirements are listed at the following site maintained by the Food and Drug Administration: **http://www.cfsan.fda.gov/~dms/lab-cons.html**. When interpreting these requirements, the government recommends that consumers become familiar with the following abbreviations before reading FDA literature:[49]

- **DVs (Daily Values):** A new dietary reference term that will appear on the food label. It is made up of two sets of references, DRVs and RDIs.

- **DRVs (Daily Reference Values):** A set of dietary references that applies to fat, saturated fat, cholesterol, carbohydrate, protein, fiber, sodium, and potassium.

- **RDIs (Reference Daily Intakes):** A set of dietary references based on the Recommended Dietary Allowances for essential vitamins and minerals

[49] Adapted from the FDA: **http://www.fda.gov/fdac/special/foodlabel/dvs.html**.

and, in selected groups, protein. The name "RDI" replaces the term "U.S. RDA."

- **RDAs (Recommended Dietary Allowances):** A set of estimated nutrient allowances established by the National Academy of Sciences. It is updated periodically to reflect current scientific knowledge.

What Are Dietary Supplements?[50]

Dietary supplements are widely available through many commercial sources, including health food stores, grocery stores, pharmacies, and by mail. Dietary supplements are provided in many forms including tablets, capsules, powders, gel-tabs, extracts, and liquids. Historically in the United States, the most prevalent type of dietary supplement was a multivitamin/mineral tablet or capsule that was available in pharmacies, either by prescription or "over the counter." Supplements containing strictly herbal preparations were less widely available. Currently in the United States, a wide array of supplement products are available, including vitamin, mineral, other nutrients, and botanical supplements as well as ingredients and extracts of animal and plant origin.

The Office of Dietary Supplements (ODS) of the National Institutes of Health is the official agency of the United States which has the expressed goal of acquiring "new knowledge to help prevent, detect, diagnose, and treat disease and disability, from the rarest genetic disorder to the common cold."[51] According to the ODS, dietary supplements can have an important impact on the prevention and management of disease and on the maintenance of health.[52] The ODS notes that considerable research on the effects of dietary supplements has been conducted in Asia and Europe where the use of plant products, in particular, has a long tradition. However, the overwhelming majority of supplements have not been studied scientifically. To explore the role of dietary supplements in the improvement of health

---

[50] This discussion has been adapted from the NIH: http://ods.od.nih.gov/whatare/whatare.html.

[51] Contact: The Office of Dietary Supplements, National Institutes of Health, Building 31, Room 1B29, 31 Center Drive, MSC 2086, Bethesda, Maryland 20892-2086, Tel: (301) 435-2920, Fax: (301) 480-1845, E-mail: **ods@nih.gov**.

[52] Adapted from **http://ods.od.nih.gov/about/about.html**. The Dietary Supplement Health and Education Act defines dietary supplements as "a product (other than tobacco) intended to supplement the diet that bears or contains one or more of the following dietary ingredients: a vitamin, mineral, amino acid, herb or other botanical; or a dietary substance for use to supplement the diet by increasing the total dietary intake; or a concentrate, metabolite, constituent, extract, or combination of any ingredient described above; and intended for ingestion in the form of a capsule, powder, softgel, or gelcap, and not represented as a conventional food or as a sole item of a meal or the diet."

care, the ODS plans, organizes, and supports conferences, workshops, and symposia on scientific topics related to dietary supplements. The ODS often works in conjunction with other NIH Institutes and Centers, other government agencies, professional organizations, and public advocacy groups.

To learn more about official information on dietary supplements, visit the ODS site at **http://ods.od.nih.gov/whatare/whatare.html**. Or contact:

> The Office of Dietary Supplements
> National Institutes of Health
> Building 31, Room 1B29
> 31 Center Drive, MSC 2086
> Bethesda, Maryland 20892-2086
> Tel: (301) 435-2920
> Fax: (301) 480-1845
> E-mail: ods@nih.gov

Finding Studies on Immune Thrombocytopenic Purpura

The NIH maintains an office dedicated to patient nutrition and diet. The National Institutes of Health's Office of Dietary Supplements (ODS) offers a searchable bibliographic database called the IBIDS (International Bibliographic Information on Dietary Supplements). The IBIDS contains over 460,000 scientific citations and summaries about dietary supplements and nutrition as well as references to published international, scientific literature on dietary supplements such as vitamins, minerals, and botanicals.[53] IBIDS is available to the public free of charge through the ODS Internet page: **http://ods.od.nih.gov/databases/ibids.html**.

After entering the search area, you have three choices: (1) IBIDS Consumer Database, (2) Full IBIDS Database, or (3) Peer Reviewed Citations Only. We recommend that you start with the Consumer Database. While you may not find references for the topics that are of most interest to you, check back periodically as this database is frequently updated. More studies can be found by searching the Full IBIDS Database. Healthcare professionals and researchers generally use the third option, which lists peer-reviewed

---

[53] Adapted from http://ods.od.nih.gov. IBIDS is produced by the Office of Dietary Supplements (ODS) at the National Institutes of Health to assist the public, healthcare providers, educators, and researchers in locating credible, scientific information on dietary supplements. IBIDS was developed and will be maintained through an interagency partnership with the Food and Nutrition Information Center of the National Agricultural Library, U.S. Department of Agriculture.

citations. In all cases, we suggest that you take advantage of the "Advanced Search" option that allows you to retrieve up to 100 fully explained references in a comprehensive format. Type "immune thrombocytopenic purpura" (or synonyms) into the search box. To narrow the search, you can also select the "Title" field.

The following information is typical of that found when using the "Full IBIDS Database" when searching using "immune thrombocytopenic purpura" (or a synonym):

- **A clinical study of patients with idiopathic thrombocytopenic purpura.**
  Author(s): Department of Internal Medicine, School of Medicine, Tokai University, Kanagawa, Japan.
  Source: Nozaki, H Tanaka, K Shimizu, M Satou, Y Tokunaga, M Usui, T Mishima, K Yonekura, S Shimizu, H Noguchi, K et al. Tokai-J-Exp-Clin-Med. 1989 June; 14(3): 231-6 0385-0005

- **A prospective, randomized trial of conventional, dose-accelerated corticosteroids and intravenous immunoglobulin in children with newly diagnosed idiopathic thrombocytopenic purpura.**
  Author(s): Department of Pediatrics, Jikei University School of Medicine, Tokyo, Japan.
  Source: Fujisawa, K Iyori, H Ohkawa, H Konishi, S Bessho, F Shirahata, A Miyazaki, S Akatsuka, J Int-J-Hematol. 2000 October; 72(3): 376-83 0925-5710

- **A rare case of arteriosclerosis obliterans without prominent risk factors complicated by idiopathic thrombocytopenic purpura. A case report.**
  Author(s): Department of Internal Medicine, Kanazawa Municipal Hospital, Kanazawa, Japan.
  Source: Yamagishi, S Ohta, M Segawa, C Abe, T Sawada, T Angiology. 1996 April; 47(4): 413-7 0003-3197

- **Acute childhood idiopathic thrombocytopenic purpura: AIEOP consensus guidelines for diagnosis and treatment.Associazione Italiana di Ematologia e Oncologia Pediatrica.**
  Author(s): Dipartimento di Biomedicina dell'Eta Evolutiva, Universita di Bari. Azienda Ospedliera Policlinico, piazza G. Cesare 11, 70124 Bari, Italy. demattia@bioetaev.uniba.it.
  Source: De Mattia, D Del Principe, D Del Vecchio, G C Jankovic, M Arrighini, A Giordano, P Menichelli, A Mori, P Zecca, M Pession, A Haematologica. 2000 April; 85(4): 420-4 0390-6078

- **Approach to the investigation and management of immune thrombocytopenic purpura in children.**
  Author(s): Department of Pediatrics, University of Toronto, Ontario, Canada.
  Source: Blanchette, V Carcao, M Semin-Hematol. 2000 July; 37(3): 299-314 0037-1963

- **Ascorbic acid for the treatment of chronic refractory idiopathic thrombocytopenic purpura (ITP).**
  Author(s): Istituto di Ematologia L. e A. Seragnoli, Universita degli Studi di Bologna, Italy.
  Source: Vianelli, N Gugliotta, L Gianni, L Belmonte, M M Catani, L Tura, S Haematologica. 1992 Jan-February; 77(1): 92-3 0390-6078

- **Autoimmune thrombocytopenic purpura.**
  Author(s): First Department of Pathology, Kansai Medical University, Osaka, Japan.
  Source: Ikehara, S Mizutani, H Kurata, Y Crit-Rev-Oncol-Hematol. 1995 April; 19(1): 33-45 1040-8428

- **Canine idiopathic thrombocytopenic purpura.**
  Author(s): Department of Clinical Sciences, College of Veterinary Medicine, Kansas State University, Manhattan 66506-5606, USA.
  Source: Lewis, D C Meyers, K M J-Vet-Intern-Med. 1996 Jul-August; 10(4): 207-18 0891-6640

- **Chronic idiopathic thrombocytopenic purpura in the elderly.**
  Author(s): Department of Hematology, Hospital General Universitario de Valencia, Spain.
  Source: Linares, M Cervero, A Colomina, P Pastor, E Lopez, A Perez, A Perella, M Carbonell, F Acta-Haematol. 1995; 93(2-4): 80-2 0001-5792

- **Clinical usefulness of vinca alkaloid slow infusion in the treatment of chronic refractory idiopathic thrombocytopenic purpura: a multicenter cooperative study.**
  Author(s): Third Department of Internal Medicine, Nippon Medical School, Tokyo.
  Source: Nomura, T Maekawa, T Uchino, H Miyazaki, T Miura, Y Abe, T Asano, S Kuriya, S Nagai, K Yawata, Y et al. Nippon-Ketsueki-Gakkai-Zasshi. 1990 February; 53(1): 98-104 0001-5806

- **Colchicine therapy in immune thrombocytopenic purpura.**
  Author(s): Department of Paediatrics, Postgraduate Institute of Medical Education and Research, Chandigarh, India.
  Source: Marwaha, R K Singh, R P Garewal, G Marwaha, N Prakash, D Sarode, R Acta-Paediatr-Scand. 1990 November; 79(11): 1118-20 0001-656X

- **Combination chemotherapy in refractory immune thrombocytopenic purpura.**
  Author(s): Department of Molecular and Experimental Medicine, Scripps Research Institute, La Jolla, CA 92037.
  Source: Figueroa, M Gehlsen, J Hammond, D Ondreyco, S Piro, L Pomeroy, T Williams, F McMillan, R N-Engl-J-Med. 1993 April 29; 328(17): 1226-9 0028-4793

- **Fc receptor blockade and immune thrombocytopenic purpura.**
  Author(s): Department of Pediatrics, New York Hospital, New York 10021, USA.
  Source: Bussel, J B Semin-Hematol. 2000 July; 37(3): 261-6 0037-1963

- **Guidelines for management of idiopathic thrombocytopenic purpura. The British Paediatric Haematology Group.**
  Author(s): Department of Paediatric Oncology, St Bartholomew's Hospital, West Smithfield, London.
  Source: Eden, O B Lilleyman, J S Arch-Dis-Child. 1992 August; 67(8): 1056-8 0003-9888

- **High-dose methylprednisolone is an alternative treatment for adults with autoimmune thrombocytopenic purpura refractory to intravenous immunoglobulins and oral corticosteroids.**
  Author(s): Laboratoire d'Immunologie Leuco-plaquettaire, Hopital Henri Mondor, Creteil, France.
  Source: Godeau, B Zini, J M Schaeffer, A Bierling, P Am-J-Hematol. 1995 April; 48(4): 282-4 0361-8609

- **Idiopathic autoimmune thrombocytopenic purpura.**
  Author(s): Duke University Medical Center, Durham, North Carolina.
  Source: Kurtzberg, J Stockman, J A Adv-Pediatr. 1994; 41111-34 0065-3101

- **Impaired suppressor function of T cells induced by autologous mixed lymphocyte reaction in patients with idiopathic thrombocytopenic purpura.**
  Author(s): Second Department of Internal Medicine, Osaka University Medical School, Japan.
  Source: Furubayashi, T Mizutani, H Take, H Honda, S Tomiyama, Y Katagiri, S Tamaki, T Tsubakio, T Kurata, Y Yonezawa, T et al. Acta-Haematol. 1992; 87(1-2): 32-6 0001-5792

- **Increased in vivo biosynthesis of prostacyclin and thromboxane A2 in chronic idiopathic thrombocytopenic purpura.**
  Author(s): Laboratoire d'Hemobiologie, Institut Pasteur, Faculte de Medecine A. Carrel, INSERM 205, Lyon, France.
  Source: Rousson, D Guichardant, M Lagarde, M Viala, J J Dechavanne, M Br-J-Haematol. 1989 July; 72(3): 402-6 0007-1048

- **Increased macrophage colony-stimulating factor levels in immune thrombocytopenic purpura.**
  Author(s): Western Pennsylvania Cancer Institute, Western Pennsylvania Hospital, Pittsburgh 15224.
  Source: Zeigler, Z R Rosenfeld, C S Nemunaitis, J J Besa, E C Shadduck, R K Blood. 1993 March 1; 81(5): 1251-4 0006-4971

- **Intravenous corticosteroids versus intravenous gammaglobulin in the treatment of acute immune thrombocytopenic purpura.**
  Author(s): Department of Pediatric Hematology-Oncology, Children's Hospital, Columbus, Ohio 43205.
  Source: Hord, J D Grossman, N J Pediatr-Hematol-Oncol. 1993 Oct-December; 10(4): 323-7 0888-0018

Federal Resources on Nutrition

In addition to the IBIDS, the United States Department of Health and Human Services (HHS) and the United States Department of Agriculture (USDA) provide many sources of information on general nutrition and health. Recommended resources include:

- healthfinder®, HHS's gateway to health information, including diet and nutrition:
  http://www.healthfinder.gov/scripts/SearchContext.asp?topic=238&page=0

- The United States Department of Agriculture's Web site dedicated to nutrition information: **www.nutrition.gov**

- The Food and Drug Administration's Web site for federal food safety information: **www.foodsafety.gov**

- The National Action Plan on Overweight and Obesity sponsored by the United States Surgeon General:
  http://www.surgeongeneral.gov/topics/obesity/

- The Center for Food Safety and Applied Nutrition has an Internet site sponsored by the Food and Drug Administration and the Department of Health and Human Services: **http://vm.cfsan.fda.gov/**

- Center for Nutrition Policy and Promotion sponsored by the United States Department of Agriculture: **http://www.usda.gov/cnpp/**

- Food and Nutrition Information Center, National Agricultural Library sponsored by the United States Department of Agriculture: **http://www.nal.usda.gov/fnic/**

- Food and Nutrition Service sponsored by the United States Department of Agriculture: **http://www.fns.usda.gov/fns/**

Additional Web Resources

A number of additional Web sites offer encyclopedic information covering food and nutrition. The following is a representative sample:

- AOL: **http://search.aol.com/cat.adp?id=174&layer=&from=subcats**

- Family Village: **http://www.familyvillage.wisc.edu/med_nutrition.html**

- Google: **http://directory.google.com/Top/Health/Nutrition/**

- Healthnotes: **http://www.thedacare.org/healthnotes/**

- Open Directory Project: **http://dmoz.org/Health/Nutrition/**

- Yahoo.com: **http://dir.yahoo.com/Health/Nutrition/**

- WebMD®Health: **http://my.webmd.com/nutrition**

- WholeHealthMD.com: **http://www.wholehealthmd.com/reflib/0,1529,,00.html**

Vocabulary Builder

The following vocabulary builder defines words used in the references in this chapter that have not been defined in previous chapters:

Alkaloid: One of a large group of nitrogenous basis substances found in plants. They are usually very bitter and many are pharmacologically active. Examples are atropine, caffeine, coniine, morphine, nicotine, quinine, strychnine. The term is also applied to synthetic substances (artificial a's) which have structures similar to plant alkaloids, such as procaine. [EU]

Biosynthesis: The building up of a chemical compound in the physiologic processes of a living organism. [EU]

Carbohydrates: A nutrient that supplies 4 calories/gram. They may be simple or complex. Simple carbohydrates are called sugars, and complex carbohydrates are called starch and fiber (cellulose). An organic compound—containing carbon, hydrogen, and oxygen—that is formed by photosynthesis in plants. Carbohydrates are heat producing and are classified as monosaccharides, disaccharides, or polysaccharides. [NIH]

Cholesterol: A soft, waxy substance manufactured by the body and used in the production of hormones, bile acid, and vitamin D and present in all parts of the body, including the nervous system, muscle, skin, liver, intestines, and heart. Blood cholesterol circulates in the bloodstream. Dietary cholesterol is found in foods of animal origin. [NIH]

Diarrhea: Passage of excessively liquid or excessively frequent stools. [NIH]

Intestinal: Pertaining to the intestine. [EU]

Iodine: A nonmetallic element of the halogen group that is represented by the atomic symbol I, atomic number 53, and atomic weight of 126.90. It is a nutritionally essential element, especially important in thyroid hormone synthesis. In solution, it has anti-infective properties and is used topically. [NIH]

Niacin: Water-soluble vitamin of the B complex occurring in various animal and plant tissues. Required by the body for the formation of coenzymes NAD and NADP. Has pellagra-curative, vasodilating, and antilipemic properties. [NIH]

Overdose: 1. to administer an excessive dose. 2. an excessive dose. [EU]

Overweight: An excess of body weight but not necessarily body fat; a body mass index of 25 to 29.9 kg/m2. [NIH]

Paediatric: Of or relating to the care and medical treatment of children; belonging to or concerned with paediatrics. [EU]

Potassium: An element that is in the alkali group of metals. It has an atomic symbol K, atomic number 19, and atomic weight 39.10. It is the chief cation in the intracellular fluid of muscle and other cells. Potassium ion is a strong electrolyte and it plays a significant role in the regulation of fluid volume and maintenance of the water-electrolyte balance. [NIH]

Riboflavin: Nutritional factor found in milk, eggs, malted barley, liver, kidney, heart, and leafy vegetables. The richest natural source is yeast. It occurs in the free form only in the retina of the eye, in whey, and in urine; its principal forms in tissues and cells are as FMN and FAD. [NIH]

Selenium: An element with the atomic symbol Se, atomic number 34, and atomic weight 78.96. It is an essential micronutrient for mammals and other animals but is toxic in large amounts. Selenium protects intracellular structures against oxidative damage. It is an essential component of glutathione peroxidase. [NIH]

Thermoregulation: Heat regulation. [EU]

Thyroxine: An amino acid of the thyroid gland which exerts a stimulating effect on thyroid metabolism. [NIH]

APPENDIX D. FINDING MEDICAL LIBRARIES

Overview

At a medical library you can find medical texts and reference books, consumer health publications, specialty newspapers and magazines, as well as medical journals. In this Appendix, we show you how to quickly find a medical library in your area.

Preparation

Before going to the library, highlight the references mentioned in this sourcebook that you find interesting. Focus on those items that are not available via the Internet, and ask the reference librarian for help with your search. He or she may know of additional resources that could be helpful to you. Most importantly, your local public library and medical libraries have Interlibrary Loan programs with the National Library of Medicine (NLM), one of the largest medical collections in the world. According to the NLM, most of the literature in the general and historical collections of the National Library of Medicine is available on interlibrary loan to any library. NLM's interlibrary loan services are only available to libraries. If you would like to access NLM medical literature, then visit a library in your area that can request the publications for you.[54]

---

[54] Adapted from the NLM: http://www.nlm.nih.gov/psd/cas/interlibrary.html.

Finding a Local Medical Library

The quickest method to locate medical libraries is to use the Internet-based directory published by the National Network of Libraries of Medicine (NN/LM). This network includes 4626 members and affiliates that provide many services to librarians, health professionals, and the public. To find a library in your area, simply visit **http://nnlm.gov/members/adv.html** or call 1-800-338-7657.

Medical Libraries Open to the Public

In addition to the NN/LM, the National Library of Medicine (NLM) lists a number of libraries that are generally open to the public and have reference facilities. The following is the NLM's list plus hyperlinks to each library Web site. These Web pages can provide information on hours of operation and other restrictions. The list below is a small sample of libraries recommended by the National Library of Medicine (sorted alphabetically by name of the U.S. state or Canadian province where the library is located):[55]

- **Alabama:** Health InfoNet of Jefferson County (Jefferson County Library Cooperative, Lister Hill Library of the Health Sciences), **http://www.uab.edu/infonet/**

- **Alabama:** Richard M. Scrushy Library (American Sports Medicine Institute), **http://www.asmi.org/LIBRARY.HTM**

- **Arizona:** Samaritan Regional Medical Center: The Learning Center (Samaritan Health System, Phoenix, Arizona), **http://www.samaritan.edu/library/bannerlibs.htm**

- **California:** Kris Kelly Health Information Center (St. Joseph Health System), **http://www.humboldt1.com/~kkhic/index.html**

- **California:** Community Health Library of Los Gatos (Community Health Library of Los Gatos), **http://www.healthlib.org/orgresources.html**

- **California:** Consumer Health Program and Services (CHIPS) (County of Los Angeles Public Library, Los Angeles County Harbor-UCLA Medical Center Library) - Carson, CA, **http://www.colapublib.org/services/chips.html**

- **California:** Gateway Health Library (Sutter Gould Medical Foundation)

- **California:** Health Library (Stanford University Medical Center), **http://www-med.stanford.edu/healthlibrary/**

---

[55] Abstracted from **http://www.nlm.nih.gov/medlineplus/libraries.html**.

- **California:** Patient Education Resource Center - Health Information and Resources (University of California, San Francisco), **http://sfghdean.ucsf.edu/barnett/PERC/default.asp**

- **California:** Redwood Health Library (Petaluma Health Care District), **http://www.phcd.org/rdwdlib.html**

- **California:** San José PlaneTree Health Library, **http://planetreesanjose.org/**

- **California:** Sutter Resource Library (Sutter Hospitals Foundation), **http://go.sutterhealth.org/comm/resc-library/sac-resources.html**

- **California:** University of California, Davis. Health Sciences Libraries

- **California:** ValleyCare Health Library & Ryan Comer Cancer Resource Center (ValleyCare Health System), **http://www.valleycare.com/library.html**

- **California:** Washington Community Health Resource Library (Washington Community Health Resource Library), **http://www.healthlibrary.org/**

- **Colorado:** William V. Gervasini Memorial Library (Exempla Healthcare), **http://www.exempla.org/conslib.htm**

- **Connecticut:** Hartford Hospital Health Science Libraries (Hartford Hospital), **http://www.harthosp.org/library/**

- **Connecticut:** Healthnet: Connecticut Consumer Health Information Center (University of Connecticut Health Center, Lyman Maynard Stowe Library), **http://library.uchc.edu/departm/hnet/**

- **Connecticut:** Waterbury Hospital Health Center Library (Waterbury Hospital), **http://www.waterburyhospital.com/library/consumer.shtml**

- **Delaware:** Consumer Health Library (Christiana Care Health System, Eugene du Pont Preventive Medicine & Rehabilitation Institute), **http://www.christianacare.org/health_guide/health_guide_pmri_health _info.cfm**

- **Delaware:** Lewis B. Flinn Library (Delaware Academy of Medicine), **http://www.delamed.org/chls.html**

- **Georgia:** Family Resource Library (Medical College of Georgia), **http://cmc.mcg.edu/kids_families/fam_resources/fam_res_lib/frl.htm**

- **Georgia:** Health Resource Center (Medical Center of Central Georgia), **http://www.mccg.org/hrc/hrchome.asp**

- **Hawaii:** Hawaii Medical Library: Consumer Health Information Service (Hawaii Medical Library), **http://hml.org/CHIS/**

- **Idaho:** DeArmond Consumer Health Library (Kootenai Medical Center), **http://www.nicon.org/DeArmond/index.htm**

- **Illinois:** Health Learning Center of Northwestern Memorial Hospital (Northwestern Memorial Hospital, Health Learning Center), **http://www.nmh.org/health_info/hlc.html**

- **Illinois:** Medical Library (OSF Saint Francis Medical Center), **http://www.osfsaintfrancis.org/general/library/**

- **Kentucky:** Medical Library - Services for Patients, Families, Students & the Public (Central Baptist Hospital), **http://www.centralbap.com/education/community/library.htm**

- **Kentucky:** University of Kentucky - Health Information Library (University of Kentucky, Chandler Medical Center, Health Information Library), **http://www.mc.uky.edu/PatientEd/**

- **Louisiana:** Alton Ochsner Medical Foundation Library (Alton Ochsner Medical Foundation), **http://www.ochsner.org/library/**

- **Louisiana:** Louisiana State University Health Sciences Center Medical Library-Shreveport, **http://lib-sh.lsuhsc.edu/**

- **Maine:** Franklin Memorial Hospital Medical Library (Franklin Memorial Hospital), **http://www.fchn.org/fmh/lib.htm**

- **Maine:** Gerrish-True Health Sciences Library (Central Maine Medical Center), **http://www.cmmc.org/library/library.html**

- **Maine:** Hadley Parrot Health Science Library (Eastern Maine Healthcare), **http://www.emh.org/hll/hpl/guide.htm**

- **Maine:** Maine Medical Center Library (Maine Medical Center), **http://www.mmc.org/library/**

- **Maine:** Parkview Hospital, **http://www.parkviewhospital.org/communit.htm#Library**

- **Maine:** Southern Maine Medical Center Health Sciences Library (Southern Maine Medical Center), **http://www.smmc.org/services/service.php3?choice=10**

- **Maine:** Stephens Memorial Hospital Health Information Library (Western Maine Health), **http://www.wmhcc.com/hil_frame.html**

- **Manitoba, Canada:** Consumer & Patient Health Information Service (University of Manitoba Libraries), **http://www.umanitoba.ca/libraries/units/health/reference/chis.html**

- **Manitoba, Canada:** J.W. Crane Memorial Library (Deer Lodge Centre), **http://www.deerlodge.mb.ca/library/libraryservices.shtml**

- **Maryland:** Health Information Center at the Wheaton Regional Library (Montgomery County, Md., Dept. of Public Libraries, Wheaton Regional Library), **http://www.mont.lib.md.us/healthinfo/hic.asp**

- **Massachusetts:** Baystate Medical Center Library (Baystate Health System), **http://www.baystatehealth.com/1024/**

- **Massachusetts:** Boston University Medical Center Alumni Medical Library (Boston University Medical Center), **http://med-libwww.bu.edu/library/lib.html**

- **Massachusetts:** Lowell General Hospital Health Sciences Library (Lowell General Hospital), **http://www.lowellgeneral.org/library/HomePageLinks/WWW.htm**

- **Massachusetts:** Paul E. Woodard Health Sciences Library (New England Baptist Hospital), **http://www.nebh.org/health_lib.asp**

- **Massachusetts:** St. Luke's Hospital Health Sciences Library (St. Luke's Hospital), **http://www.southcoast.org/library/**

- **Massachusetts:** Treadwell Library Consumer Health Reference Center (Massachusetts General Hospital), **http://www.mgh.harvard.edu/library/chrcindex.html**

- **Massachusetts:** UMass HealthNet (University of Massachusetts Medical School), **http://healthnet.umassmed.edu/**

- **Michigan:** Botsford General Hospital Library - Consumer Health (Botsford General Hospital, Library & Internet Services), **http://www.botsfordlibrary.org/consumer.htm**

- **Michigan:** Helen DeRoy Medical Library (Providence Hospital and Medical Centers), **http://www.providence-hospital.org/library/**

- **Michigan:** Marquette General Hospital - Consumer Health Library (Marquette General Hospital, Health Information Center), **http://www.mgh.org/center.html**

- **Michigan:** Patient Education Resouce Center - University of Michigan Cancer Center (University of Michigan Comprehensive Cancer Center), **http://www.cancer.med.umich.edu/learn/leares.htm**

- **Michigan:** Sladen Library & Center for Health Information Resources - Consumer Health Information, **http://www.sladen.hfhs.org/library/consumer/index.html**

- **Montana:** Center for Health Information (St. Patrick Hospital and Health Sciences Center), **http://www.saintpatrick.org/chi/librarydetail.php3?ID=41**

- **National:** Consumer Health Library Directory (Medical Library Association, Consumer and Patient Health Information Section), **http://caphis.mlanet.org/directory/index.html**

- **National:** National Network of Libraries of Medicine (National Library of Medicine) - provides library services for health professionals in the United States who do not have access to a medical library, **http://nnlm.gov/**

- **National:** NN/LM List of Libraries Serving the Public (National Network of Libraries of Medicine), **http://nnlm.gov/members/**

- **Nevada:** Health Science Library, West Charleston Library (Las Vegas Clark County Library District), **http://www.lvccld.org/special_collections/medical/index.htm**

- **New Hampshire:** Dartmouth Biomedical Libraries (Dartmouth College Library), **http://www.dartmouth.edu/~biomed/resources.htmld/conshealth.htmld/**

- **New Jersey:** Consumer Health Library (Rahway Hospital), **http://www.rahwayhospital.com/library.htm**

- **New Jersey:** Dr. Walter Phillips Health Sciences Library (Englewood Hospital and Medical Center), **http://www.englewoodhospital.com/links/index.htm**

- **New Jersey:** Meland Foundation (Englewood Hospital and Medical Center), **http://www.geocities.com/ResearchTriangle/9360/**

- **New York:** Choices in Health Information (New York Public Library) - NLM Consumer Pilot Project participant, **http://www.nypl.org/branch/health/links.html**

- **New York:** Health Information Center (Upstate Medical University, State University of New York), **http://www.upstate.edu/library/hic/**

- **New York:** Health Sciences Library (Long Island Jewish Medical Center), **http://www.lij.edu/library/library.html**

- **New York:** ViaHealth Medical Library (Rochester General Hospital), **http://www.nyam.org/library/**

- **Ohio:** Consumer Health Library (Akron General Medical Center, Medical & Consumer Health Library), **http://www.akrongeneral.org/hwlibrary.htm**

- **Oklahoma:** Saint Francis Health System Patient/Family Resource Center (Saint Francis Health System), **http://www.sfh-tulsa.com/patientfamilycenter/default.asp**

- **Oregon:** Planetree Health Resource Center (Mid-Columbia Medical Center), **http://www.mcmc.net/phrc/**

- **Pennsylvania:** Community Health Information Library (Milton S. Hershey Medical Center), **http://www.hmc.psu.edu/commhealth/**

- **Pennsylvania:** Community Health Resource Library (Geisinger Medical Center), **http://www.geisinger.edu/education/commlib.shtml**

- **Pennsylvania:** HealthInfo Library (Moses Taylor Hospital), **http://www.mth.org/healthwellness.html**

- **Pennsylvania:** Hopwood Library (University of Pittsburgh, Health Sciences Library System), **http://www.hsls.pitt.edu/chi/hhrcinfo.html**

- **Pennsylvania:** Koop Community Health Information Center (College of Physicians of Philadelphia), **http://www.collphyphil.org/kooppg1.shtml**

- **Pennsylvania:** Learning Resources Center - Medical Library (Susquehanna Health System), **http://www.shscares.org/services/lrc/index.asp**

- **Pennsylvania:** Medical Library (UPMC Health System), **http://www.upmc.edu/passavant/library.htm**

- **Quebec, Canada:** Medical Library (Montreal General Hospital), **http://ww2.mcgill.ca/mghlib/**

- **South Dakota:** Rapid City Regional Hospital - Health Information Center (Rapid City Regional Hospital, Health Information Center), **http://www.rcrh.org/education/LibraryResourcesConsumers.htm**

- **Texas:** Houston HealthWays (Houston Academy of Medicine-Texas Medical Center Library), **http://hhw.library.tmc.edu/**

- **Texas:** Matustik Family Resource Center (Cook Children's Health Care System), **http://www.cookchildrens.com/Matustik_Library.html**

- **Washington:** Community Health Library (Kittitas Valley Community Hospital), **http://www.kvch.com/**

- **Washington:** Southwest Washington Medical Center Library (Southwest Washington Medical Center), **http://www.swmedctr.com/Home/**

Appendix E. NIH Consensus Statement on Platelet Transfusion Therapy

Overview

NIH Consensus Development Conferences are convened to evaluate available scientific information and resolve safety and efficacy issues related to biomedical technology. The resultant NIH Consensus Statements are intended to advance understanding of the technology or issue in question and to be useful to health professionals and the public.[56] Each NIH consensus statement is the product of an independent, non-Federal panel of experts and is based on the panel's assessment of medical knowledge available at the time the statement was written. Therefore, a consensus statement provides a "snapshot in time" of the state of knowledge of the conference topic.

The NIH makes the following caveat: "When reading or downloading NIH consensus statements, keep in mind that new knowledge is inevitably accumulating through medical research. Nevertheless, each NIH consensus statement is retained on this website in its original form as a record of the NIH Consensus Development Program."[57] The following concensus statement was posted on the NIH site and not indicated as "out of date" in March 2002. It was originally published, however, in October, 1986.[58]

---

[56] This paragraph has been adapted from the NIH:
http://odp.od.nih.gov/consensus/cons/cons.htm.
[57] Adapted from the NIH: **http://odp.od.nih.gov/consensus/cons/consdate.htm**.
[58] **Platelet Transfusion Therapy**. NIH Consens Statement Online 1986 Oct 6-8 [cited 2002 February 19];6(7):1-6. **http://consensus.nih.gov/cons/059/059_statement.htm**.

What Is Platelet Transfusion Therapy?

In the past, patients with chronic thrombocytopenia died of hemorrhage with distressingly predictable frequency. The increased use of platelet transfusions during the past 15 years has prevented most such deaths. Furthermore, this therapy has made it possible to treat patients with drugs who have otherwise fatal disorders that temporarily suppress platelet production. With this great benefit, however, have come complex problems. Transfused platelets can transmit fatal diseases and can elicit an immune response in recipients, so that further transfusions are no longer effective. Although platelet therapy has contributed greatly to the management of patients with many diseases such as acute leukemia and aplastic anemia, serious questions have emerged regarding its use in patients undergoing cardiac surgery and in other circumstances. The prophylactic administration of platelets is also controversial, and there is uncertainty as to the platelet levels that predispose thrombocytopenic patients to hemorrhage and as to the effectiveness of modalities other than platelets in the prevention of bleeding. The relative merits of the various methods for obtaining and storing platelets remain unclear. The advantages and disadvantages of platelets obtained from multiple and single donors require evaluation.

To resolve these issues, the National Heart, Lung, and Blood Institute, National Institutes of Health (NIH), the Center for Drugs and Biologics of the Food and Drug Administration, and the NIH Office of Medical Applications of Research convened a Consensus Development Conference on Platelet Transfusion Therapy on October 6-8, 1986. At a 1 1/2-day series of presentations by experts in the field, a consensus panel drawn from the medical professions, blood banking organizations, and the general public considered the evidence. The panel agreed on answers to the following key questions:

- What are the appropriate indications for platelet transfusion?

- What products are available, and what are their relative merits?

- What are the risks associated with platelet transfusion?

- What are the most important directions for future research?

What Are the Appropriate Indications for Platelet Transfusion?

Despite the obvious advantages of platelet transfusion therapy, there is concern that platelets are sometimes given to patients who do not really need them, are given too often to patients who do need them, and occasionally are given in insufficient quantities when treatment is urgently required. Clinical decisions regarding platelet transfusion are hampered by an insufficient number of properly controlled trials, by imprecise methods of evaluating clinical need, and by uncertain methods for measuring effects.

The platelet levels that predispose thrombocytopenic patients to hemorrhage and the efficacy of therapeutic modalities other than transfusion are not well defined. It is apparent that factors other than the platelet count must also be considered in deciding when to transfuse. The efficacy of transfused platelets may be altered by other abnormalities in the recipient such as uremia, concomitant coagulation disorders, or medications. The rate and direction of change in platelet count must also be considered.

Active Bleeding

Patients with thrombocytopenia or an abnormality of platelet function or both who have significant bleeding should receive platelets if the platelet disorder is likely to be causing or contributing to the bleeding. It is sometimes difficult to make this judgment clinically. It is unlikely that a patient with a platelet count of 50,000 per microliter or higher will benefit from a platelet transfusion if thrombocytopenia is the sole abnormality. If the disorder is one of function, reliance must be placed on some test of platelet function, such as the template bleeding time. A bleeding time of less than twice the upper limit of normal is usually not an indication for transfusion of platelets, unless there are other conditions that interfere with hemostasis. Patients with thrombocytopenia resulting from platelet destruction or splenic pooling may require more intensive transfusion therapy than those with marrow hypoplasia.

Prophylaxis

The patient with severe thrombocytopenia may benefit from prophylactic administration of platelets. This is particularly true of patients with a temporary thrombocytopenia consequent to myelosuppressive therapy. It is common practice to use a preselected level of thrombocytopenia to decide when to transfuse platelets prophylactically. The value of 20,000 platelets per microliter is often used. This figure is based on older studies with potential defects as judged by current knowledge. Recent evidence suggests that this number might safely be lower for some patients based on clinical judgment and close observation. A problem with selecting specific concentrations is the lack of reproducibility and the variability of platelet counts at low levels.

Patients with chronic thrombocytopenia caused by impaired platelet production (e.g., aplastic anemia, myelodysplastic disorders) generally do not require routine platelet transfusions. Patients with accelerated destruction but active production of platelets (e.g., immune thrombocytopenic purpura) have relatively less bleeding at a given platelet count than patients with hypoplastic platelet disorders. Thus, platelet transfusions are rarely needed in these conditions. Other appropriate medical and surgical therapy is usually effective. Preparation for invasive procedures in thrombocytopenic or thrombocytopathic patients might include prophylactic administration of platelets. In many instances there are associated disorders of coagulation or platelet function that cannot be completely corrected, as is common in patients with advanced hepatic or renal insufficiency. In such patients, transfusion of platelets may be necessary, especially for procedures in which hemostasis cannot be assessed by direct observation. Transfusion of enough platelets to correct the bleeding time to the normal range is logical, but there are few, if any, pertinent studies. A similar approach may be justified for patients threatened with hemorrhage in the central nervous system or other sites in which a small amount of bleeding could be critical.

Massive Transfusion

Dilutional thrombocytopenia occurs in patients receiving multiple tranfusions to replace blood lost through hemorrhage and may lead to generalized microvascular bleeding. The degree of dilution is usually predictable. Following replacement of one blood volume, 35 to 40 percent of the platelets usually remain. Thrombocytopenia is accentuated in the presence of accelerated platelet destruction, which sometimes occurs in such patients, mandating performance of platelet counts as a guide to platelet therapy. The majority of patients who receive rapid replacement of one to two blood volumes do not develop microvascular bleeding as a result of thrombocytopenia. Therefore, platelets should not be administered in the absence of documented thrombocytopenia and clinically abnormal bleeding.

Cardiac Surgery

Controlled prospective studies examining postoperative blood loss and outcome have demonstrated no correlation between platelet counts and bleeding following cardiopulmonary bypass and no detectable benefit from the prophylactic administration of platelets to such patients. The vast majority of such patients have some degree of thrombocytopenia, prolongation of the bleeding time, and continued slow bleeding. With an expected pattern of bleeding, thrombocytopenia alone is not an indication for platelet transfusion. There is no justification for prophylactic platelet administration in patients undergoing open heart surgery.

Newborns

Because of the special nature of neonatal requirements for blood and blood products as well as dosages, these issues were not addressed specifically in this report. Nonetheless, efforts should be exerted to continue to avoid undue exposure to multiple donor sources.

What Products Are Available? What Are Their Relative Merits?

Platelets can be harvested from single donors by plateletapheresis or separated from whole blood, with pooling of cells from multiple donors to achieve a therapeutic dose. Single-donor platelets[59] can be obtained from random donors or from donors selected on the basis of HLA compatibility. Local conditions and practices often influence the choice among these alternatives, but there are identifiable advantages and disadvantages of each product that should be considered. These include availability, potential for disease transmission, and potential for alloimmunization.

Products

Since each single-donor apheresis collection provides the equivalent of the platelets obtained from five to eight whole blood donations, this product exposes a patient to fewer donors and offers potential advantages over the multiple-donor product: less exposure to infectious agents and reduced likelihood of alloimmunization. However, there is no evidence that single-donor platelets are either more or less effective than multiple-donor concentrates in patients who have not become alloimmunized.

---

[59] The term single-donor platelets is used to mean platelets obtained by apheresis from a single donor. The number of platelets obtained is approximately equal to the number of platelets obtained from five to eight whole-blood donations.

A major advantage of multiple-donor platelets is that they are in relatively plentiful supply, having been derived from conventional whole-blood donations. Moreover, they can be stored for 5 days, assuring a stable community resource. Storage time for single-donor platelets depends on the method used for harvesting; in some cases, the product must be used within 24 hours.

Certain organizational and logistical considerations influence the choice of platelets from random or HLA-matched single donors. Donation of platelets by apheresis requires a greater donor commitment than does whole-blood donation, as well as sophisticated equipment and highly trained personnel. Even where enough donors are available, the complexity of the procedure as currently employed can make its routine use infeasible. However, HLA-matched single-donor products are currently the most effective therapy for patients who have become refractory to unselected single-donor or multiple-donor platelets.

Storage

Platelets are normally stored at 20° C to 24° C, with constant agitation for up to 5 days. Although platelets stored at 4° C are a licensed product, they are now rarely used because of their reduced survival and function after transfusion.

Platelets can be frozen to extend their storage period. Since patients who have become refractory to platelet transfusions during one course of chemotherapy will usually be difficult to treat during subsequent periods of chemotherapy-induced hypoplasia, their anticipated need can be met by the cryopreservation of autologous platelets obtained by apheresis during a remission. The low yield and high cost of cryopreserved platelets have limited their use in other conditions.

Dosage

The therapeutic dose of platelets is affected by the patient's pretransfusion platelet count and blood volume, as well as by associated clinical conditions. The common practice of transfusing multiple-donor platelets at a dose of 1 unit per 10 kg body weight, or of transfusing a concentrate obtained from one apheresis donor, is a reasonable starting point for platelet therapy in the adult patient. The effect of a transfusion should be judged by the clinical result and the platelet count obtained 1 hour later. These measures plus later platelet counts as indicated can also provide guidance for further treatment.

A standard 170 micron filter is recommended for the administration of platelets. Filters of smaller pore size are not indicated.

Adjunctive Therapies

Several agents have been used in addition to, or in place of, platelets in the treatment of thrombocytopenia resulting from impaired production or platelet dysfunction. Epsilon-aminocaproic acid (EACA) and prednisone have been considered useful for the treatment of these conditions by some clinicians, but there are no satisfactory studies that support their regular use. In uremia, bleeding responds in many cases to treatment with cryoprecipitate or desmopressin (DDAVP), and platelet transfusions can be avoided.

What Are the Risks Associated with Platelet Transfusion Therapy?

The major risks associated with platelet transfusion are alloimmunization and infection. Rarely, platelet transfusions cause graft-versus-host disease.

Alloimmunization and the Refractory State

When platelet-reactive antibodies are induced by transfusion, platelets subsequently administered often fail to produce a therapeutic benefit. A poor response to transfused platelets also can be caused by splenomegaly, fever, sepsis, disseminated intravascular coagulation, nonviable platelets, and other conditions. Alloimmunization to platelet antigens is common in patients who have received repeated transfusions. However, an appreciable number of patients fail to form platelet-reactive antibodies for reasons that are not clear. There is no well-defined relationship between the number of donor exposures and the extent of antibody formation, although one study suggests a lower incidence of alloimmunization in patients exposed to platelets derived by apheresis from fewer donors. Alloimmunization to the HLA-A and HLA-B antigens is encountered most frequently. Evidence indicates that leukocytes, present in routinely prepared platelet concentrates, provoke HLA-antibody formation more readily than platelets.

The failure of HLA-matched platelets to elevate the platelet count after transfusion to some alloimmunized patients suggests that antibodies reactive with non-HLA, platelet-specific antigens can cause destruction of transfused platelets. Circulating immune complexes have also been implicated. ABO compatibility between donor and recipient is of minor importance in platelet transfusion therapy in most adults. Administration of ABO incompatible platelets is an acceptable transfusion practice. The possibility of Rh immunization by red cells contained in platelet concentrates should be considered in female recipients.

Various strategies have been proposed to cope with the therapeutic problems presented by alloimmunized, thrombocytopenic patients. Administration of leukocyte-poor blood products to patients likely to require continuing transfusion support has been advocated to reduce the frequency of alloimmunization, but the feasibility and effectiveness of this strategy have not been conclusively demonstrated. The same is true of the prospective use of platelets from single donors. New approaches to this problem, still in an experimental stage, are treatment of platelet concentrates with ultraviolet light to abolish the immunogenicity of contaminating leukocytes and the transfusion of soluble, class I HLA antigens to induce active tolerance.

Various techniques have been used to improve the effectiveness of platelets in alloimmunized patients. The most feasible of these is the transfusion of HLA-matched platelets from family members or unrelated persons. If not available locally, matched platelets can sometimes be obtained from regional blood centers with access to large panels of HLA-typed donors. Only about two-thirds of HLA-matched platelet transfusions given to alloimmunized patients are effective. Newer immunologic techniques appear capable of predicting transfusion response in such patients with an 80 percent to 90 percent certainty. These assays are available in only a few centers and are not yet applicable to standard transfusion practice. High-dose intravenous immunoglobulin therapy, splenectomy, and removal of alloantibodies by plasmapheresis may be of marginal benefit but cannot be recommended for routine use.

Infection

Infections transmitted by platelet transfusions are similar to those associated with other blood components. These are of special concern because platelet transfusions often are prepared by pooling concentrates from multiple donors and are given in large numbers to immunocompromised patients.

With agents infrequently present in donated blood such as the human immunodeficiency virus (HIV), the risk of infection is roughly proportional to the number of donor exposures. As with other blood products, agents causing most of the serious infections are the non-A, non-B hepatitis virus(es), hepatitis B virus, cytomegalovirus, and HIV. The risk of disease transmission with blood transfusion varies geographically and among donor populations but appears to be decreasing nationally because of newly implemented test methods and donor screening policies.

An unusual, but sometimes fatal, complication of platelet transfusion is infusion of bacteria that have proliferated in concentrates stored at 20° C to 24° C. Physicians should be aware of this complication and be prepared to administer antibiotics and supportive measures. Attempts should be made to identify the source of the contamination in all such cases.

Graft-Versus-Host Disease

Graft-versus-host disease is a rare complication of platelet transfusions that can be prevented by gamma irradiation of concentrates prior to transfusion to patients who have undergone bone marrow transplantation or have other forms of immunodeficiency.

Directions for Future Research

Research should be directed toward the following[60]:

Recipient-Related Issues

- Development of a practical test that predicts the likelihood of clinically significant platelet-related bleeding.

- Controlled clinical trials to evaluate strategies for prophylactic use of platelets in patients with disorders of platelet production.

- Evaluation of pharmacologic approaches designed to reduce platelet requirements.

---

[60] Priorities are not implied in this sequence.

Product-Related Issues

- Development of better techniques to harvest platelets with minimal contamination with other blood components.

- Better methods of platelet preservation.

- Practical means for detecting ineffective units and bacterial contamination prior to transfusion.

- Better characterization of platelet alloantigens and the development of practical methods to detect platelet alloantibodies and select compatible donors.

- Effective means to prevent alloimmunization and to manage the alloimmunized patient.

- Development of methods and strategies to lessen the incidence of transfusion-transmitted diseases.

- Monitoring of the patterns of platelet use.

Donor-Related Issues

- Assessment of the long-term effects of repeated plateletapheresis.

- Identification of factors leading to successful recruitment of plateletapheresis donors.

Platelet use is controlled locally and determined largely by existing practice. Attempts to alter platelet use frequently have been ineffective. The most successful attempts can be attributed to a strong local proponent of appropriate transfusion practices. Ongoing collaborative efforts, including component therapy workshops involving clinicians, blood bank directors, and members of hospital transfusion committees, can do much to alter existing practices. Increased attention to the risks and benefits of component therapy in medical schools and teaching hospitals also may change the use of platelet concentrates. When appropriate, information regarding potential risks and benefits of platelets and other blood products should be made available to patients who receive those products. Monitoring the patterns of platelet use on a continuing basis will provide a means for evaluating the impact of those strategies and a basis for suggesting additional or alternative approaches.

Conclusions

In this document, the panel has made a number of observations and recommendations based on information presented at this conference relating to the indications for platelet transfusion, products available, and associated risks. We believe platelets are overused in some conditions. An example is the prophylactic use of platelets in open heart surgery, a practice the panel believes is unwarranted. Some of the uncertainty surrounding platelet transfusion practices is related to the lack of methods for predicting which patients are at risk to bleed and the effectiveness of various platelet preparations. We recommend research initiatives to provide better guidelines for transfusion practice.

More basic research to elucidate the role of platelets in hemostasis is needed. In addition, better information on current platelet transfusion practices, obtained through a surveillance system at a national level, would be of great benefit as an educational tool. Efforts to overcome the problems associated with alloimmunization to platelets are imperative. A major step in this regard would be the establishment of a national network to facilitate transfusion of HLA-matched platelets to selected patients. Infections transmitted by platelet transfusions remain a major concern. Elimination of bacterial growth in platelet concentrates stored at room temperatures warrants special attention.

Vocabulary Builder

Antibiotics: Substances produced by microorganisms that can inhibit or suppress the growth of other microorganisms. [NIH]

Cardiopulmonary: Pertaining to the heart and lungs. [EU]

Contamination: The soiling or pollution by inferior material, as by the introduction of organisms into a wound, or sewage into a stream. [EU]

Cryopreservation: Preservation of cells, tissues, organs, or embryos by freezing. In histological preparations, cryopreservation or cryofixation is used to maintain the existing form, structure, and chemical composition of all the constituent elements of the specimens. [NIH]

Hemostasis: The process which spontaneously arrests the flow of blood from vessels carrying blood under pressure. It is accomplished by contraction of the vessels, adhesion and aggregation of formed blood elements, and the process of blood or plasma coagulation. [NIH]

Hepatitis: Inflammation of the liver. [EU]

Hypoplasia: Incomplete development or underdevelopment of an organ or tissue. [EU]

Intravascular: Within a vessel or vessels. [EU]

Pharmacologic: Pertaining to pharmacology or to the properties and reactions of drugs. [EU]

Postoperative: Occurring after a surgical operation. [EU]

Prophylaxis: The prevention of disease; preventive treatment. [EU]

Proportional: Being in proportion : corresponding in size, degree, or intensity, having the same or a constant ratio; of, relating to, or used in determining proportions. [EU]

Remission: A diminution or abatement of the symptoms of a disease; also the period during which such diminution occurs. [EU]

Surgical: Of, pertaining to, or correctable by surgery. [EU]

APPENDIX F. MORE ON AUTOIMMUNE DISEASES

Overview[61]

The word "auto" is the Greek word for self. The immune system is a complicated network of cells and cell components (called molecules) that normally work to defend the body and eliminate infections caused by bacteria, viruses, and other invading microbes. If a person has an autoimmune disease, the immune system mistakenly attacks self, targeting the cells, tissues, and organs of a person's own body. A collection of immune system cells and molecules at a target site is broadly referred to as inflammation.

There are many different autoimmune diseases, and they can each affect the body in different ways. For example, the autoimmune reaction is directed against the brain in multiple sclerosis and the gut in Crohn's disease. In other autoimmune diseases such as systemic lupus erythematosus (lupus), affected tissues and organs may vary among individuals with the same disease. One person with lupus may have affected skin and joints whereas another may have affected skin, kidney, and lungs. Ultimately, damage to certain tissues by the immune system may be permanent, as with destruction of insulin-producing cells of the pancreas in Type 1 diabetes mellitus.

Who Is Affected by Autoimmune Diseases?

Many of the autoimmune diseases are rare. As a group, however, autoimmune diseases afflict millions of Americans. Most autoimmune

---

[61] Adapted from the National Institute of Allergy and Infectious Diseases (NIAID): **http://www.niaid.nih.gov/publications/autoimmune/contents.htm**.

diseases strike women more often than men; in particular, they affect women of working age and during their childbearing years.

Some autoimmune diseases occur more frequently in certain minority populations. For example, lupus is more common in African-American and Hispanic women than in Caucasian women of European ancestry. Rheumatoid arthritis and scleroderma affect a higher percentage of residents in some Native American communities than in the general U.S. population. Thus, the social, economic, and health impact from autoimmune diseases is far-reaching and extends not only to family but also to employers, co-workers, and friends.

What Are the Causes of Autoimmune Diseases?

Are they contagious? No autoimmune disease has ever been shown to be contagious or "catching." Autoimmune diseases do not spread to other people like infections. They are not related to AIDS, nor are they a type of cancer.

Are they inherited? The genes people inherit contribute to their susceptibility for developing an autoimmune disease. Certain diseases such as psoriasis can occur among several members of the same family. This suggests that a specific gene or set of genes predisposes a family member to psoriasis. In addition, individual family members with autoimmune diseases may inherit and share a set of abnormal genes, although they may develop different autoimmune diseases. For example, one first cousin may have lupus, another may have dermatomyositis, and one of their mothers may have rheumatoid arthritis.

Examples of Autoimmune Diseases by System

Nervous system:

- Multiple sclerosis

- Myasthenia gravis

- Autoimmune neuropathies such as Guillain-Barré

- Autoimmune uveitis

Gastrointestinal system:

- Crohn's Disease

- Ulcerative colitis
- Primary biliary cirrhosis
- Autoimmune hepatitis

Endocrine glands:
- Type 1 or immune-mediated diabetes mellitus
- Hashimoto's thyroiditis
- Grave's Disease

Blood:
- Autoimmune hemolytic anemia
- Pernicious anemia
- Immune thrombocytopenic purpura
- Autoimmune oophoritis and orchitis
- Autoimmune disease of the adrenal gland

Blood vessels:
- Temporal arteritis
- Anti-phospholipid syndrome
- Vasculitides such as Wegener's granulomatosis
- Behcet's disease

Multiple organs including the musculoskeletal system[62]:
- Rheumatoid arthritis
- Systemic lupus erythematosus
- Scleroderma
- Polymyositis, dermatomyositis
- Spondyloarthropathies such as ankylosing spondylitis
- Sjogren's syndrome

---

[62] These diseases are also called connective tissue (muscle, skeleton, tendons, fascia, etc.) diseases.

Skin:

- Psoriasis
- Dermatitis herpetiformis
- Pemphigus vulgaris
- Vitiligo

The development of an autoimmune disease may be influenced by the genes a person inherits together with the way the person's immune system responds to certain triggers or environmental influences.

What May Influence the Development of Autoimmune Diseases?

Some autoimmune diseases are known to begin or worsen with certain triggers such as viral infections. Sunlight not only acts as a trigger for lupus but can worsen the course of the disease. It is important to be aware of the factors that can be avoided to help prevent or minimize the amount of damage from the autoimmune disease. Other less understood influences affecting the immune system and the course of autoimmune diseases include aging, chronic stress, hormones, and pregnancy.

How Does the Immune System Work?

The immune system defends the body from attack by invaders recognized as foreign. It is an extraordinarily complex system that relies on an elaborate and dynamic communications network that exists among the many different kinds of immune system cells that patrol the body. At the heart of the system is the ability to recognize and respond to substances called antigens whether they are infectious agents or part of the body (self antigens).

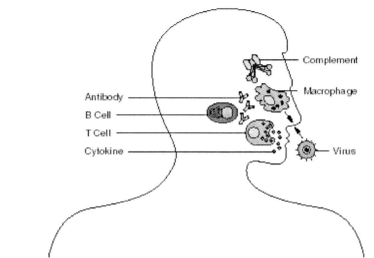

Cells and molecules of the immune system protect the nose from attack by a virus.

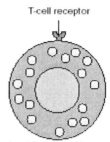

T cell (lymphocyte) with a T-cell receptor on its surface.

T and B Cells

Most immune system cells are white blood cells, of which there are many types. Lymphocytes are one type of white blood cell, and two major classes of lymphocytes are T cells and B cells. T cells are critical immune system cells that help to destroy infected cells and coordinate the overall immune response. The T cell has a molecule on its surface called the T-cell receptor. This receptor interacts with molecules called MHC (major histocompatibility complex). MHC molecules are on the surfaces of most other cells of the body and help T cells recognize antigen fragments. B cells are best known for making antibodies. An antibody binds to an antigen and marks the antigen for destruction by other immune system cells. Other types of white blood cells include macrophages and neutrophils.

Macrophages and Neutrophils

Macrophages and neutrophils circulate in the blood and survey the body for foreign substances. When they find foreign antigens, such as bacteria, they engulf and destroy them. Macrophages and neutrophils destroy foreign antigens by making toxic molecules such as reactive oxygen intermediate molecules. If production of these toxic molecules continues unchecked, not only are the foreign antigens destroyed, but tissues surrounding the macrophages and neutrophils are also destroyed. For example, in individuals with the autoimmune disease called Wegener's granulomatosis, overactive macrophages and neutrophils that invade blood vessels produce many toxic molecules and contribute to damage of the blood vessels. In rheumatoid arthritis, reactive oxygen intermediate molecules and other toxic molecules are made by overproductive macrophages and neutrophils invading the joints. The toxic molecules contribute to inflammation, which is observed as warmth and swelling, and participate in damage to the joint.

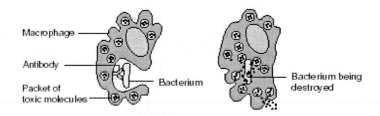

A macrophage engulfing a bacterium and releasing packets of toxic molecules (reactive oxygen intermediates) that break down and destroy the bacterium.

MHC and Co-Stimulatory Molecules

MHC molecules are found on all cell surfaces and are an active part of the body's defense team. For example, when a virus infects a cell, a MHC molecule binds to a piece of a virus (antigen) and displays the antigen on the cell's surface. Cells that have the capability of displaying antigen with MHC are called antigen-presenting cells. Each MHC molecule that displays an antigen is recognized by a matching or compatible T-cell receptor. Thus, an antigen-presenting cell is able to communicate with a T cell about what may be occurring inside the cell.

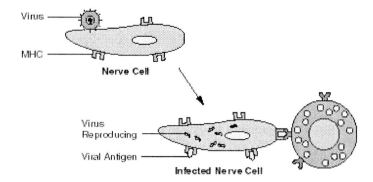

Upper left: a virus attacking a nerve cell. Lower right: a T cell with a T-cell receptor recognizing a piece of a virus (antigen) on the MHC of the infected nerve cell.

However, for the T cell to respond to a foreign antigen on the MHC, another molecule on the antigen-presenting cell must send a second signal to the T cell. A corresponding molecule on the surface of the T cells recognizes the second signal. These two secondary molecules of the antigen-presenting cell and the T cell are called co-stimulatory molecules. There are several different sets of co-stimulatory molecules that can participate in the interaction of antigen-presenting cell with a T cell.

Once the MHC and the T-cell receptor interact, and the co-stimulatory molecules interact, there are several possible paths that the T cell may take. These include T cell activation, tolerance, or T cell death. The subsequent steps depend in part on which co-stimulatory molecules interact and how well they interact. Because these interactions are so critical to the response of the immune system, researchers are intensively studying them to find new therapies that could control or stop the immune system attack on self tissues and organs.

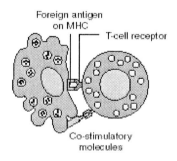

An antigen-presenting cell (for example, a macrophage) with a foreign antigen on its MHC is recognized by a T-cell receptor. In addition, co-stimulatory molecules on the antigen-presenting cell and the T cell interact.

Cytokines and Chemokines

One way T cells can respond after the interaction of the MHC and the T-cell receptor, and the interaction of the co-stimulatory molecules, is to secrete cytokines and chemokines. Cytokines are proteins that may cause surrounding immune system cells to become activated, grow, or die. They also may influence non-immune system tissues. For example, some cytokines may contribute to the thickening of the skin that occurs in people with scleroderma.

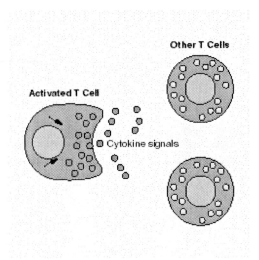

After the antigen-presenting cell and T cell interact through the MHC, T-cell receptor and co-stimumlatory and molecules, the T cell becomes activated, sending cytokine signals to other cells.

Chemokines are small cytokine molecules that attract cells of the immune system. Overproduction of chemokines contributes to the invasion and inflammation of the target organ, which occurs in autoimmune diseases. For example, overproduction of chemokines in the joints of people with rheumatoid arthritis may result in invasion of the joint space by destructive immune system cells such as macrophages, neutrophils, and T cells.

Antibodies

B cells are another critical type of immune system cell. They participate in the removal of foreign antigens from the body by using a surface molecule to bind the antigen or by making specific antibodies that can search out and destroy specific foreign antigens. However, the B cell can only make antibodies when it receives the appropriate command signal from a T cell. Once the T cell signals the B cell with a type of cytokine that acts as a messenger molecule, the B cell is able to produce a unique antibody that targets a particular antigen.

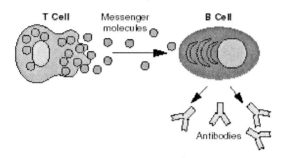

A T cell sends messenger molecules, e.g. cytokines, to the B cell, which allows the B cell to start making antibodies.

Autoantibodies

In some autoimmune diseases, B cells mistakenly make antibodies against tissues of the body (self antigens) instead of foreign antigens. Occasionally, these autoantibodies either interfere with the normal function of the tissues or initiate destruction of the tissues. People with myasthenia gravis experience muscle weakness because autoantibodies attack a part of the nerve that stimulates muscle movement. In the skin disease pemphigus vulgaris, autoantibodies are misdirected against cells in the skin. The accumulation of antibodies in the skin activates other molecules and cells to break down, resulting in skin blisters.

Immune Complexes and the Complement System

When many antibodies are bound to antigens in the bloodstream, they form a large lattice network called an immune complex. Immune complexes are harmful when they accumulate and initiate inflammation within small blood vessels that nourish tissues. Immune complexes, immune cells, and inflammatory molecules can block blood flow and ultimately destroy organs such as the kidney. This can occur in people with systemic lupus erythematosus.

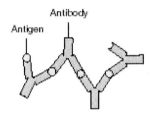

A large immune complex.

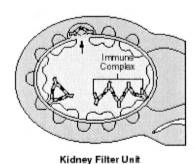

Kidney Filter Unit

If immune complexes accumulate in the kidney, they may promote movement of other inflammatory cells and molecules into the kidney.

A group of specialized molecules that form the complement system helps to remove immune complexes. The different types of molecules of the complement system, which are found in the bloodstream and on the surfaces of cells, make immune complexes more soluble. Complement molecules prevent formation and reduce the size of immune complexes so they do not accumulate in the wrong places (organs and tissues of the body). Rarely, some people inherit defective genes for a complement molecule from their parents. Because these individuals cannot make a normal amount or type of complement molecule, their immune systems are unable to prevent immune complexes from being deposited in different tissues and organs. These people develop a disease that is not autoimmune but resembles lupus erythematosus.

Genetic Factors

Genetic factors can affect an individual's immune system and its responses to foreign antigens in several ways. Genes determine the variety of MHC molecules that individuals carry on their cells. Genes also influence the potential array of T-cell receptors present on T cells. In fact, some MHC genes are associated with autoimmune diseases. However, genes are not the only factors involved in determining a person's susceptibility to an autoimmune disease. For example, some individuals who carry disease-associated MHC molecules on their cells will not develop an autoimmune disease.

How Are Autoimmune Diseases Diagnosed?

The diagnosis of an autoimmune disease is based on an individual's symptoms, findings from a physical examination, and results from laboratory tests. Autoimmune diseases can be difficult to diagnose, particularly early in the course of the disease. Symptoms of many autoimmune diseases—such as fatigue—are nonspecific. Laboratory test results may help but are often inadequate to confirm a diagnosis.

If an individual has skeletal symptoms such as joint pain and a positive but nonspecific lab test, she or he may be diagnosed with the confusing name of early or "undifferentiated" connective tissue disease. In this case, a physician may want the patient to return frequently for follow up. The early phase of disease may be a very frustrating time for both the patient and physician. On the other hand, symptoms may be short-lived, and inconclusive laboratory tests may amount to nothing of a serious nature.

In some cases, a specific diagnosis can be made. A diagnosis shortly after onset of a patient's symptoms will allow for early aggressive medical therapy; and for some diseases, patients will respond completely to treatments if the reason for their symptoms is discovered early in the course of their disease.

Although autoimmune diseases are chronic, the course they take is unpredictable. A doctor cannot foresee what will happen to the patient based on how the disease starts. Patients should be monitored closely by their doctors so environmental factors or triggers that may worsen the disease can be discussed and avoided and new medical therapy can be started as soon as possible. Frequent visits to a doctor are important in order for the physician to manage complex treatment regimens and watch for medication side effects.

How Are Autoimmune Diseases Treated?

Autoimmune diseases are often chronic, requiring lifelong care and monitoring, even when the person may look or feel well. Currently, few autoimmune diseases can be cured or made to "disappear" with treatment. However, many people with these diseases can live normal lives when they receive appropriate medical care.

Physicians most often help patients manage the consequences of inflammation caused by the autoimmune disease. For example, in people with Type 1 diabetes, physicians prescribe insulin to control blood sugar levels so that elevated blood sugar will not damage the kidneys, eyes, blood vessels, and nerves. However, the goal of scientific research is to prevent inflammation from causing destruction of the insulin-producing cells of the pancreas, which are necessary to control blood sugars.

On the other hand, in some diseases such as lupus or rheumatoid arthritis, medication can occasionally slow or stop the immune system's destruction of the kidneys or joints. Medications or therapies that slow or suppress the immune system response in an attempt to stop the inflammation involved in the autoimmune attack are called immunosuppressive medications. These drugs include corticosteroids (prednisone), methotrexate, cyclophosphamide, azathioprine, and cyclosporin. Unfortunately, these medications also suppress the ability of the immune system to fight infection and have other potentially serious side effects.

In some people, a limited number of immuno-suppressive medications may result in disease remission. Remission is the medical term used for "disappearance" of a disease for a significant amount of time. Even if their disease goes into remission, patients are rarely able to discontinue medications. The possibility that the disease may restart when medication is discontinued must be balanced with the long-term side effects from the immunosuppressive medication.

A current goal in caring for patients with autoimmune diseases is to find treatments that produce remissions with fewer side effects. Much research is focused on developing therapies that target various steps in the immune response. New approaches such as therapeutic antibodies against specific T cell molecules may produce fewer long-term side effects than the chemotherapies that now are routinely used.

Ultimately, medical science is striving to design therapies that prevent autoimmune diseases. To this end, a significant amount of time and resources are spent studying the immune system and pathways of inflammation.

What Are Some Examples of Autoimmune Diseases?

Rheumatoid Arthritis

In people with rheumatoid arthritis, the immune system predominantly targets the lining (synovium) that covers various joints. Inflammation of the synovium is usually symmetrical (occurring equally on both sides of the body) and causes pain, swelling, and stiffness of the joints. These features distinguish rheumatoid arthritis from osteoarthritis, which is a more common and degenerative "wear-and-tear" arthritis.

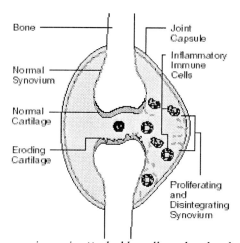

An inflamed joint – the synovium – is attacked by cells and molecules of the immune system.

Currently available therapy focuses on reducing inflammation of the joints with anti-inflammatory or immunosuppresssive medications. Sometimes, the immune system may also target the lung, blood vessels, or eye; occasionally patients may also develop symptoms of other autoimmune diseases such as Sjogren's the inflammation, itching, and scaling. For more severe cases, oral medications are used. Psoriasis is common and may affect more than 2 out of 100 Americans. Psoriasis often runs in families.

Multiple Sclerosis

Multiple sclerosis is a disease in which the immune system targets nerve tissues of the central nervous system. Most commonly, damage to the central nervous system occurs intermittently, allowing a person to lead a fairly normal life. At the other extreme, the symptoms may become constant, resulting in a progressive disease with possible blindness, paralysis, and premature death. Some medications such as beta interferon are helpful to people with the intermittent form of multiple sclerosis.

In young adults, multiple sclerosis is the most common disabling disease of the nervous system. Multiple sclerosis afflicts 1 in 700 people in this country. Researchers continue to search for triggers of the disease.

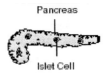

Immune-Mediated or Type 1 Diabetes Mellitus

Type 1 diabetes mellitus results from autoimmune destruction of the insulin-producing cells of the pancreas. Insulin is required by the body to keep the blood sugar (glucose) level under control. High levels of glucose are responsible for the symptoms and the complications of the disease. However, most of the insulin-producing cells are destroyed before the patient develops symptoms of diabetes. Symptoms include fatigue, frequent urination, increased thirst, and possible sudden confusion.

Type 1 diabetes mellitus is usually diagnosed before the age of 30 and may be diagnosed as early as the first month of life. Together with Type 2 diabetes (not considered an autoimmune disease), diabetes mellitus is the leading cause of kidney damage, loss of eyesight, and leg amputation. Close control of sugar levels decreases the rate at which these events occur. There is a genetic predisposition to Type 1 diabetes, which occurs in 1 out of 800 people in the United States. Among individuals who have a close relative with Type 1 diabetes, those at high risk for developing disease can be identified. Efforts are now under way to evaluate prevention strategies for these family members at risk.

Inflammatory Bowel Diseases

This medical term is used for both Crohn's disease and ulcerative colitis, two diseases in which the immune system attacks the gut (intestine). Patients may have diarrhea, nausea, vomiting, abdominal cramps, and pain that can be difficult to control. Illness in afflicted individuals can result from intestinal inflammation and from side effects of the drugs used for the disease. For example, daily use of high-dose corticosteroid (prednisone) therapy, which is needed to control severe symptoms of Crohn's disease, can predispose patients to infections, bone thinning (osteoporosis), and fractures. For patients with ulcerative colitis, surgical removal of the lower intestine (colon) will eliminate the disease and their increased risk for colon cancer. More than 1 in 500 Americans has some type of inflammatory bowel disease.

Systemic Lupus Erythematosus

Patients with systemic lupus erythematosus most commonly experience profound fatigue, rashes, and joint pains. In severe cases, the immune system may attack and damage several organs such as the kidney, brain, or lung. For many individuals, symptoms and damage from the disease can be controlled with available anti-inflammatory medications. However, if a patient is not closely monitored, the side effects from the medications can be quite serious. Lupus occurs in 1 out of 2,000 Americans and in as many as 1 in 250 young, African-American women.

Psoriasis

Psoriasis is an immune system disorder that affects the skin, and occasionally the eyes, nails, and joints. Psoriasis may affect very small areas of skin or cover the entire body with a buildup of red scales called plaques. The plaques are of different sizes, shapes, and severity and may be painful as well as unattractive. Bacterial infections and pressure or trauma to the skin can aggravate psoriasis. Most treatments focus on topical skin care to relieve the inflammation, itching, and scaling. For more severe cases, oral medications are used. Psoriasis is common and may affect more than 2 out of 100 Americans. Psoriasis often runs in families.

Scleroderma

This autoimmune disease results in thickening of the skin and blood vessels. Almost every patient with scleroderma has Raynaud's, which is a spasm of the blood vessels of the fingers and toes. Symptoms of Raynaud's include increased sensitivity of the fingers and toes to the cold, changes in skin color, pain, and occasionally ulcers of the fingertips or toes. In people with scleroderma, thickening of skin and blood vessels can result in loss of movement and shortness of breath or, more rarely, in kidney, heart, or lung failure. The estimated number of people with any type of scleroderma varies from study to study but may range from 1 to 4 affected individuals for every 10,000 Americans (or as many as 1 out of 2500 individuals).

Autoimmune Thyroid Diseases

Hashimoto's thyroiditis and Grave's disease result from immune system destruction or stimulation of thyroid tissue. Symptoms of low (hypo-) or overactive (hyper-) thyroid function are nonspecific and can develop slowly or suddenly; these include fatigue, nervousness, cold or heat intolerance, weakness, changes in hair texture or amount, and weight gain or loss. The diagnosis of thyroid disease is readily made with appropriate laboratory tests.

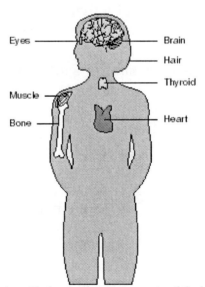

The thyroid gland affect many parts of the body.

The symptoms of hypothyroidism are controlled with replacement thyroid hormone pills; however, complications from over- or under-replacement of the hormone can occur. Treatment of hyperthyroidism requires long-term anti-thyroid drug therapy or destruction of the thyroid gland with radioactive iodine or surgery. Both of these treatment approaches carry certain risks and long-term side effects. Autoimmune thyroid diseases afflict as many as 4 out of 100 women and are frequently found in families where there are other autoimmune diseases.

What Research Is Under Way on Autoimmune Diseases?

The National Institute of Allergy and Infectious Diseases (NIAID) supports research studies on the function of the immune system in various diseases. A basic understanding of the human immune system is central to the understanding of the development of an autoimmune disease (disease pathogenesis). Scientists searching for ways to prevent and treat autoimmune disease are studying disease pathogenesis and investigating new ways to modify the immune system.

Specifically, investigators supported by NIAID are focusing on: 1) studies of the immune system during the progression of an autoimmune disease; 2) analysis of the influence of genetics on autoimmune disease expression and progression; 3) the role of infectious agents in autoimmune diseases; 4) studies of animal models of autoimmune diseases; and 5) the effects of therapeutic intervention on the immune system in an autoimmune disease.

In addition, studies of a specific autoimmune disease such as multiple sclerosis can provide new and additional insights into the pathogenesis of autoimmune diseases affecting other organ systems. Therefore, NIAID also supports studies on specific autoimmune diseases in cooperation with other Institutes of the National Institutes of Health that focus on organ-specific autoimmune diseases.

Resources

National Institutes of Health (NIH) Resources

The following NIH components support medical research and/or provide information on varying aspects of autoimmune diseases.

National Institute of Allergy and Infectious Diseases
Office of Communications
Bldg. 31/Rm. 7A50
31 Center Drive, MSC 2520
Bethesda, MD 20892-2520
(301) 496-5717
http://www.niaid.nih.gov/publications/
http://www.niaid.nih.gov/clintrials/default.htm (for clinical trials
information)

National Institute of Arthritis and Musculoskeletal and Skin Diseases
Information Clearinghouse/NIH
1 AMS Circle
Bethesda, MD 20892-3675
Fast Facts: (301) 881-2731 (to receive information by fax)
Clearinghouse: (301) 495-4484
http://www.nih.gov/niams/healthinfo/

National Institute of Diabetes and Digestive and Kidney Diseases
(NIDDK)
Information Clearinghouse
1 Information Way
Bethesda, MD 20892-3560
Diabetes, Digestive, and Kidney Diseases Information:
(301) 654-3810

NIDDK Information Office (Thyroid Diseases)
Bldg. 31/Rm. 9A04
31 Center Drive
Bethesda, MD 20892-3560
(301) 496-3583
http://www.niddk.nih.gov

National Institute of Neurological Disorders and Stroke
Office of Scientific and Health Reports
P.O. Box 5801
Bethesda, MD 20824
(301) 496-5751
http://www.ninds.nih.gov/

NIH Clinical Center
Patient Recruitment and Referral Center—for specific NIH clinical trials information
4 West Drive, MSC 2655
Quarters 15 D-2
Bethesda, MD 20892-2655
(301) 411-1222
http://clinicalstudies.info.nih.gov/referring_patient.html

Office of Rare Diseases, NIH
Bldg. 31/Rm. 1B03
31 Center Drive
Bethesda, MD 20892
(301) 402-4336
http://rarediseases.info.nih.gov/ord/

Other Resources Sponsored by the Department of Health and Human Services

National Health Information Center
(800) 336-4797 or (301) 565-4167
Health Finder: **http://www.healthfinder.gov**

Combined Health Information Database
http://chid.nih.gov

Private Sector Organizations

The following list is astarting point for additional information on autoimmune diseases. Many of the organizations have extensive educational resources, local chapters, and support groups. The Internet Web site of many organizations can refer you to other disease-oriented groups (for example, the Arthritis Foundation has alink to the Lupus Foundation).

American Autoimmune Related Diseases Association
15475 Gratiot Avenue
Detroit, MI 48205
(800) 598-4668 or (313) 371-8600
http://www.aarda.org/

American Diabetes Association
1660 Duke Street
Alexandria, VA 22314
(800) 232-3472 or (703) 549-1500
http://www.diabetes.org/

American Liver Foundation
1425 Pompton Avenue
Cedar Grove, NJ 07009
(800) 233-0179 and (973) 256-2550

American Thyroid Association Montefiore Medical Center
111 East 210th Street
Bronx, NY 10467
Fax: (718) 882-6085
http://www.thyroid.org/

Arthritis Foundation
1650 Bluegrass Lakes Pkwy.
Alpharetta, GA 30009
(800) 283-7800 or (800) 207-8633
http://www.arthritis.org

Crohn's and Colitis Foundation of America
National Headquarters
386 Park Avenue South, 17th Floor
New York, NY 10016-8804
(800) 932-2423
(800) 343-3637 (Warehouse)
http://www.ccfa.org

Juvenile Diabetes Foundation International
120 Wall Street
New York, NY 10005-4001
(800) JDF-CURE or (800) 533-2873
http://www.jdf.org

Lupus Foundation of America
1300 Piccard Drive, Suite 200
Rockville, MD 20850-4303
(800) 558-0121 and (301) 670-9292
http://www.lupus.org/

Myasthenia Gravis Foundation of America
222 S. Riverside Plaza, Suite 1540
Chicago, IL 60606
(800) 541-5454 or (312) 258-0522
http://www.myasthenia.org/

Myositis Association of America
755 Cantrell Avenue
Suite C
Harrisonburg, VA 22801
(540) 433-7686
http://www.myositis.org

National Adrenal Diseases Foundation
505 Northern Boulevard
Great Neck, NY 11021
(516) 487-4992
http://www.medhelp.org/nadf/

National Alopecia Areata Foundation
710 CStreet, Suite 11
San Rafael, CA 94901-3853
or
P.O. Box 150760
San Rafael, CA 94915-0760
(415) 456-4644
Fax: (415) 456-4274
http://www.alopeciaareata.com

National Multiple Sclerosis Society
733 Third Avenue, 6th Floor
New York, NY 10017-3288
(800) 344-4867 or (212) 986-3240
Fax: (212) 986-7981
http://www.nmss.org
e-mail: ire@nmss.org

National Organization for Rare Disorders
P.O. Box 8923
New Fairfield, CT 06812-1783
(800) 999-6673
http://www.rarediseases.org/

National Psoriasis Foundation
6600 SW 92nd Avenue, Suite 300
Portland, OR 97223
(800) 723-9166 or (503) 244-7404
http://www.psoriasis.org

National Sjogren's Syndrome Association
5815 N. Black Canyon Highway, Suite 103
Phoenix, AZ 85015-2200
(602) 433-9844
http://www.sjogrens.org

National Vitiligo Foundation
P.O. Box 6337
Tyler, TX 75703
(903) 531-0074
Fax: (903) 531-9767
http://www.nvfi.org

Sjogren's Syndrome Foundation
333 N. Broadway
Jericho, NY 11753
1-800-4-SJOGRENS or (516) 933-6365
http://www.sjogrens.com

Spondylitis Association of America
P.O. Box 5872
Sherman Oaks, CA 91413
(800) 777-8189 or (888) 777-1594
http://www.spondylitis.org/

The S.L.E. Foundation
149 Madison Avenue, Suite 205
New York, NY 10016
(800) 745-8787
http://www.lupus.org

United Scleroderma Foundation
89 Newbury Street, Suite 201
Danvers, MA 01923
800) 722-HOPE
Fax: (978) 750-9902
http://www.scleroderma.org

Wegener's Foundation
3705 South George Mason Drive, Suite 1813
Falls Church, VA 22041
(703) 931-5852

Wegener's Granulomatosis Support Group
P.O. Box 28660
Kansas City, MO 64188-8668
(800) 277-9474
Fax: (816) 436-8211
http://www.wgsg.org/

ONLINE GLOSSARIES

The Internet provides access to a number of free-to-use medical dictionaries and glossaries. The National Library of Medicine has compiled the following list of online dictionaries:

- ADAM Medical Encyclopedia (A.D.A.M., Inc.), comprehensive medical reference: **http://www.nlm.nih.gov/medlineplus/encyclopedia.html**

- MedicineNet.com Medical Dictionary (MedicineNet, Inc.): **http://www.medterms.com/Script/Main/hp.asp**

- Merriam-Webster Medical Dictionary (Inteli-Health, Inc.): **http://www.intelihealth.com/IH/**

- Multilingual Glossary of Technical and Popular Medical Terms in Eight European Languages (European Commission) - Danish, Dutch, English, French, German, Italian, Portuguese, and Spanish: **http://allserv.rug.ac.be/~rvdstich/eugloss/welcome.html**

- On-line Medical Dictionary (CancerWEB): **http://www.graylab.ac.uk/omd/**

- Technology Glossary (National Library of Medicine) - Health Care Technology: **http://www.nlm.nih.gov/nichsr/ta101/ta10108.htm**

- Terms and Definitions (Office of Rare Diseases): **http://rarediseases.info.nih.gov/ord/glossary_a-e.html**

Beyond these, MEDLINEplus contains a very user-friendly encyclopedia covering every aspect of medicine (licensed from A.D.A.M., Inc.). The ADAM Medical Encyclopedia Web site address is **http://www.nlm.nih.gov/medlineplus/encyclopedia.html**. ADAM is also available on commercial Web sites such as Web MD (**http://my.webmd.com/adam/asset/adam_disease_articles/a_to_z/a**) and drkoop.com (**http://www.drkoop.com/**). Topics of interest can be researched by using keywords before continuing elsewhere, as these basic definitions and concepts will be useful in more advanced areas of research. You may choose to print various pages specifically relating to immune thrombocytopenic purpura and keep them on file. The NIH, in particular, suggests that patients with immune thrombocytopenic purpura visit the following Web sites in the ADAM Medical Encyclopedia:

- **Basic Guidelines for Immune Thrombocytopenic Purpura**

  Idiopathic thrombocytopenic purpura (ITP)
  Web site:
  http://www.nlm.nih.gov/medlineplus/ency/article/000535.htm

- **Signs & Symptoms for Immune Thrombocytopenic Purpura**

  Bleeding disorder
  Web site:
  http://www.nlm.nih.gov/medlineplus/ency/article/001304.htm

  Bruising
  Web site:
  http://www.nlm.nih.gov/medlineplus/ency/article/003235.htm

  Enlarged spleen
  Web site:
  http://www.nlm.nih.gov/medlineplus/ency/article/003276.htm

  Pinpoint red spots
  Web site:
  http://www.nlm.nih.gov/medlineplus/ency/article/003235.htm

  Rash
  Web site:
  http://www.nlm.nih.gov/medlineplus/ency/article/003220.htm

- **Diagnostics and Tests for Immune Thrombocytopenic Purpura**

  Biopsy
  Web site:
  http://www.nlm.nih.gov/medlineplus/ency/article/003416.htm

  Bone marrow aspiration
  Web site:
  http://www.nlm.nih.gov/medlineplus/ency/article/003658.htm

  CBC
  Web site:
  http://www.nlm.nih.gov/medlineplus/ency/article/003642.htm

Platelet aggregation test
Web site:
http://www.nlm.nih.gov/medlineplus/ency/article/003669.htm

Platelet associated antibodies
Web site:
http://www.nlm.nih.gov/medlineplus/ency/article/003552.htm

Platelet count
Web site:
http://www.nlm.nih.gov/medlineplus/ency/article/003647.htm

Platelets
Web site:
http://www.nlm.nih.gov/medlineplus/ency/article/003647.htm

PT
Web site:
http://www.nlm.nih.gov/medlineplus/ency/article/003652.htm

PTT
Web site:
http://www.nlm.nih.gov/medlineplus/ency/article/003653.htm

- **Nutrition for Immune Thrombocytopenic Purpura**

Protein
Web site:
http://www.nlm.nih.gov/medlineplus/ency/article/002467.htm

- **Surgery and Procedures for Immune Thrombocytopenic Purpura**

Splenectomy
Web site:
http://www.nlm.nih.gov/medlineplus/ency/article/002944.htm

- **Background Topics for Immune Thrombocytopenic Purpura**

Antibodies
Web site:
http://www.nlm.nih.gov/medlineplus/ency/article/002223.htm

Bleeding
Web site:
http://www.nlm.nih.gov/medlineplus/ency/article/000045.htm

Chronic
Web site:
http://www.nlm.nih.gov/medlineplus/ency/article/002312.htm

Incidence
Web site:
http://www.nlm.nih.gov/medlineplus/ency/article/002387.htm

Physical examination
Web site:
http://www.nlm.nih.gov/medlineplus/ency/article/002274.htm

Online Dictionary Directories

The following are additional online directories compiled by the National
Library of Medicine, including a number of specialized medical dictionaries
and glossaries:

- Medical Dictionaries: Medical & Biological (World Health Organization):
  http://www.who.int/hlt/virtuallibrary/English/diction.htm#Medical

- MEL-Michigan Electronic Library List of Online Health and Medical
  Dictionaries (Michigan Electronic Library):
  http://mel.lib.mi.us/health/health-dictionaries.html

- Patient Education: Glossaries (DMOZ Open Directory Project):
  http://dmoz.org/Health/Education/Patient_Education/Glossaries/

- Web of Online Dictionaries (Bucknell University):
  http://www.yourdictionary.com/diction5.html#medicine

IMMUNE THROMBOCYTOPENIC PURPURA GLOSSARY

The following is a complete glossary of terms used in this sourcebook. The definitions are derived from official public sources including the National Institutes of Health [NIH] and the European Union [EU]. After this glossary, we list a number of additional hardbound and electronic glossaries and dictionaries that you may wish to consult.

ACTH: Adrenocorticotropic hormone. [EU]

Adenosine: A nucleoside that is composed of adenine and d-ribose. Adenosine or adenosine derivatives play many important biological roles in addition to being components of DNA and RNA. Adenosine itself is a neurotransmitter. [NIH]

Adjuvant: A substance which aids another, such as an auxiliary remedy; in immunology, nonspecific stimulator (e.g., BCG vaccine) of the immune response. [EU]

Agonist: In anatomy, a prime mover. In pharmacology, a drug that has affinity for and stimulates physiologic activity at cell receptors normally stimulated by naturally occurring substances. [EU]

Alkaloid: One of a large group of nitrogenous basis substances found in plants. They are usually very bitter and many are pharmacologically active. Examples are atropine, caffeine, coniine, morphine, nicotine, quinine, strychnine. The term is also applied to synthetic substances (artificial a's) which have structures similar to plant alkaloids, such as procaine. [EU]

Anatomical: Pertaining to anatomy, or to the structure of the organism. [EU]

Anemia: A reduction in the number of circulating erythrocytes or in the quantity of hemoglobin. [NIH]

Anergy: Absence of immune response to particular substances. [NIH]

Antibody: An immunoglobulin molecule that has a specific amino acid sequence by virtue of which it interacts only with the antigen that induced its synthesis in cells of the lymphoid series (especially plasma cells), or with antigen closely related to it. Antibodies are classified according to their ode of action as agglutinins, bacteriolysins, haemolysins, opsonins, precipitins, etc. [EU]

Antigen: Any substance which is capable, under appropriate conditions, of inducing a specific immune response and of reacting with the products of that response, that is, with specific antibody or specifically sensitized T-lymphocytes, or both. Antigens may be soluble substances, such as toxins and foreign proteins, or particulate, such as bacteria and tissue cells; however, only the portion of the protein or polysaccharide molecule known as the antigenic determinant (q.v.) combines with antibody or a specific receptor on a lymphocyte. Abbreviated Ag. [EU]

Aplasia: Lack of development of an organ or tissue, or of the cellular products from an organ or tissue. [EU]

Arrestin: A 48-Kd protein of the outer segment of the retinal rods and a component of the phototransduction cascade. Arrestin quenches G-protein activation by binding to phosphorylated photolyzed rhodopsin. Arrestin causes experimental autoimmune uveitis when injected into laboratory animals. [NIH]

Arteritis: Inflammation of an artery. [NIH]

Assay: Determination of the amount of a particular constituent of a mixture, or of the biological or pharmacological potency of a drug. [EU]

Atopic: Pertaining to an atopen or to atopy; allergic. [EU]

Auricular: Pertaining to an auricle or to the ear, and, formerly, to an atrium of the heart. [EU]

Autoimmunity: Process whereby the immune system reacts against the body's own tissues. Autoimmunity may produce or be caused by autoimmune diseases. [NIH]

Biopsy: The removal and examination, usually microscopic, of tissue from the living body, performed to establish precise diagnosis. [EU]

Biosynthesis: The building up of a chemical compound in the physiologic processes of a living organism. [EU]

Candidiasis: Infection with a fungus of the genus Candida. It is usually a superficial infection of the moist cutaneous areas of the body, and is generally caused by C. albicans; it most commonly involves the skin (dermatocandidiasis), oral mucous membranes (thrush, def. 1), respiratory tract (bronchocandidiasis), and vagina (vaginitis). Rarely there is a systemic infection or endocarditis. Called also moniliasis, candidosis, oidiomycosis, and formerly blastodendriosis. [EU]

Carbohydrates: A nutrient that supplies 4 calories/gram. They may be simple or complex. Simple carbohydrates are called sugars, and complex carbohydrates are called starch and fiber (cellulose). An organic compound — containing carbon, hydrogen, and oxygen— that is formed by photosynthesis in plants. Carbohydrates are heat producing and are classified as monosaccharides, disaccharides, or polysaccharides. [NIH]

Cardiac: Pertaining to the heart. [EU]

Cardiopulmonary: Pertaining to the heart and lungs. [EU]

Cell: Basic subunit of every living organism; the simplest unit that can exist as an independent living system. [NIH]

Cervical: Pertaining to the neck, or to the neck of any organ or structure. [EU]

Cheilitis: Inflammation of the lips. It is of various etiologies and degrees of pathology. [NIH]

Chemotherapy: The treatment of disease by means of chemicals that have a specific toxic effect upon the disease - producing microorganisms or that selectively destroy cancerous tissue. [EU]

Cholesterol: A soft, waxy substance manufactured by the body and used in the production of hormones, bile acid, and vitamin D and present in all parts of the body, including the nervous system, muscle, skin, liver, intestines, and heart. Blood cholesterol circulates in the bloodstream. Dietary cholesterol is found in foods of animal origin. [NIH]

Chronic: Of long duration; frequently recurring. [NIH]

Chymotrypsin: A serine endopeptidase secreted by the pancreas as its zymogen, chymotrypsinogen and carried in the pancreatic juice to the duodenum where it is activated by trypsin. It selectively cleaves aromatic amino acids on the carboxyl side. [NIH]

Cocaine: An alkaloid ester extracted from the leaves of plants including coca. It is a local anesthetic and vasoconstrictor and is clinically used for that purpose, particularly in the eye, ear, nose, and throat. It also has powerful central nervous system effects similar to the amphetamines and is a drug of abuse. Cocaine, like amphetamines, acts by multiple mechanisms on brain catecholaminergic neurons; the mechanism of its reinforcing effects is thought to involve inhibition of dopamine uptake. [NIH]

Contamination: The soiling or pollution by inferior material, as by the introduction of organisms into a wound, or sewage into a stream. [EU]

Contraception: The prevention of conception or impregnation. [EU]

Corticosteroids: Drugs that mimic the action of a group of hormones produced by adrenal glands; they are anti-inflammatory and act as bronchodilators. [NIH]

Cryopreservation: Preservation of cells, tissues, organs, or embryos by freezing. In histological preparations, cryopreservation or cryofixation is used to maintain the existing form, structure, and chemical composition of all the constituent elements of the specimens. [NIH]

Cyclophosphamide: Precursor of an alkylating nitrogen mustard antineoplastic and immunosuppressive agent that must be activated in the liver to form the active aldophosphamide. It is used in the treatment of lymphomas, leukemias, etc. Its side effect, alopecia, has been made use of in defleecing sheep. Cyclophosphamide may also cause sterility, birth defects, mutations, and cancer. [NIH]

Cytokines: Non-antibody proteins secreted by inflammatory leukocytes and some non-leukocytic cells, that act as intercellular mediators. They differ from classical hormones in that they are produced by a number of tissue or cell types rather than by specialized glands. They generally act locally in a paracrine or autocrine rather than endocrine manner. [NIH]

Cytomegalovirus: A genus of the family herpesviridae, subfamily betaherpesvirinae, infecting the salivary glands, liver, spleen, lungs, eyes, and other organs, in which they produce characteristically enlarged cells with intranuclear inclusions. Infection with Cytomegalovirus is also seen as an opportunistic infection in AIDS. [NIH]

Danazol: A synthetic steroid with antigonadotropic and anti-estrogenic activities that acts as an anterior pituitary suppressant by inhibiting the pituitary output of gonadotropins. It possesses some androgenic properties. Danazol has been used in the treatment of endometriosis and some benign breast disorders. [NIH]

Degenerative: Undergoing degeneration : tending to degenerate; having the character of or involving degeneration; causing or tending to cause degeneration. [EU]

Dementia: An acquired organic mental disorder with loss of intellectual abilities of sufficient severity to interfere with social or occupational functioning. The dysfunction is multifaceted and involves memory, behavior, personality, judgment, attention, spatial relations, language, abstract thought, and other executive functions. The intellectual decline is usually progressive, and initially spares the level of consciousness. [NIH]

Dendritic: 1. branched like a tree. 2. pertaining to or possessing dendrites. [EU]

Diarrhea: Passage of excessively liquid or excessively frequent stools. [NIH]

Digestion: The process of breakdown of food for metabolism and use by the body. [NIH]

Ecchymosis: A small haemorrhagic spot, larger than a petechia, in the skin or mucous membrane forming a nonelevated, rounded or irregular, blue or purplish patch. [EU]

Efficacy: The extent to which a specific intervention, procedure, regimen, or service produces a beneficial result under ideal conditions. Ideally, the determination of efficacy is based on the results of a randomized control trial. [NIH]

Endothelium: The layer of epithelial cells that lines the cavities of the heart and of the blood and lymph vessels, and the serous cavities of the body, originating from the mesoderm. [EU]

Endotoxin: Toxin from cell walls of bacteria. [NIH]

Eosinophils: Granular leukocytes with a nucleus that usually has two lobes connected by a slender thread of chromatin, and cytoplasm containing coarse, round granules that are uniform in size and stainable by eosin. [NIH]

Epithelium: The covering of internal and external surfaces of the body, including the lining of vessels and other small cavities. It consists of cells joined by small amounts of cementing substances. Epithelium is classified into types on the basis of the number of layers deep and the shape of the superficial cells. [EU]

Epitopes: Sites on an antigen that interact with specific antibodies. [NIH]

Etoposide: A semisynthetic derivative of podophyllotoxin that exhibits antitumor activity. Etoposide inhibits DNA synthesis by forming a complex with topoisomerase II and DNA. This complex induces breaks in double stranded DNA and prevents repair by topoisomerase II binding. Accumulated breaks in DNA prevent entry into the mitotic phase of cell division, and lead to cell death. Etoposide acts primarily in the G2 and S phases of the cell cycle. [NIH]

Fatigue: The state of weariness following a period of exertion, mental or physical, characterized by a decreased capacity for work and reduced efficiency to respond to stimuli. [NIH]

Gangrene: Death of tissue, usually in considerable mass and generally associated with loss of vascular (nutritive) supply and followed by bacterial invasion and putrefaction. [EU]

Gestation: The period of development of the young in viviparous animals, from the time of fertilization of the ovum until birth. [EU]

Gingivitis: Inflammation of the gingivae. Gingivitis associated with bony changes is referred to as periodontitis. Called also oulitis and ulitis. [EU]

Glomerular: Pertaining to or of the nature of a glomerulus, especially a renal glomerulus. [EU]

Glomerulonephritis: A variety of nephritis characterized by inflammation of the capillary loops in the glomeruli of the kidney. It occurs in acute, subacute, and chronic forms and may be secondary to haemolytic streptococcal infection. Evidence also supports possible immune or autoimmune mechanisms. [EU]

Haemostasis: The arrest of bleeding, either by the physiological properties of vasoconstriction and coagulation or by surgical means. [EU]

Hematology: A subspecialty of internal medicine concerned with morphology, physiology, and pathology of the blood and blood-forming tissues. [NIH]

Hematoma: An extravasation of blood localized in an organ, space, or tissue. [NIH]

Hemorrhage: Bleeding or escape of blood from a vessel. [NIH]

Hemostasis: The process which spontaneously arrests the flow of blood from vessels carrying blood under pressure. It is accomplished by contraction of the vessels, adhesion and aggregation of formed blood elements, and the process of blood or plasma coagulation. [NIH]

Hepatic: Pertaining to the liver. [EU]

Hepatitis: Inflammation of the liver. [EU]

Herpes: Any inflammatory skin disease caused by a herpesvirus and characterized by the formation of clusters of small vesicles. When used alone, the term may refer to herpes simplex or to herpes zoster. [EU]

Homeostasis: A tendency to stability in the normal body states (internal environment) of the organism. It is achieved by a system of control mechanisms activated by negative feedback; e.g. a high level of carbon dioxide in extracellular fluid triggers increased pulmonary ventilation, which in turn causes a decrease in carbon dioxide concentration. [EU]

Humoral: Of, relating to, proceeding from, or involving a bodily humour - now often used of endocrine factors as opposed to neural or somatic. [EU]

Hybridomas: Cells artificially created by fusion of activated lymphocytes with neoplastic cells. The resulting hybrid cells are cloned and produce pure or "monoclonal" antibodies or T-cell products, identical to those produced by the immunologically competent parent, and continually grow and divide as the neoplastic parent. [NIH]

Hypersensitivity: A state of altered reactivity in which the body reacts with an exaggerated immune response to a foreign substance. Hypersensitivity reactions are classified as immediate or delayed, types I and IV, respectively, in the Gell and Coombs classification (q.v.) of immune responses. [EU]

Hypoplasia: Incomplete development or underdevelopment of an organ or tissue. [EU]

Idiopathic: Results from an unknown cause. [NIH]

Immunity: The condition of being immune; the protection against infectious disease conferred either by the immune response generated by immunization or previous infection or by other nonimmunologic factors (innate i.). [EU]

Immunization: Protection from disease by administering vaccines that induce the body to form antibodies against infectious agents. [NIH]

Immunodiffusion: Technique involving the diffusion of antigen or antibody through a semisolid medium, usually agar or agarose gel, with the result being a precipitin reaction. [NIH]

Induction: The act or process of inducing or causing to occur, especially the production of a specific morphogenetic effect in the developing embryo through the influence of evocators or organizers, or the production of anaesthesia or unconsciousness by use of appropriate agents. [EU]

Infiltration: The diffusion or accumulation in a tissue or cells of substances not normal to it or in amounts of the normal. Also, the material so accumulated. [EU]

Inflammation: Response of the body tissues to injury; typical signs are swelling, redness, and pain. [NIH]

Influenza: An acute viral infection involving the respiratory tract. It is marked by inflammation of the nasal mucosa, the pharynx, and conjunctiva, and by headache and severe, often generalized, myalgia. [NIH]

Infusion: The therapeutic introduction of a fluid other than blood, as saline solution, solution, into a vein. [EU]

Intestinal: Pertaining to the intestine. [EU]

Intravascular: Within a vessel or vessels. [EU]

Intravenous: Within a vein or veins. [EU]

Iodine: A nonmetallic element of the halogen group that is represented by the atomic symbol I, atomic number 53, and atomic weight of 126.90. It is a nutritionally essential element, especially important in thyroid hormone synthesis. In solution, it has anti-infective properties and is used topically. [NIH]

Kinetic: Pertaining to or producing motion. [EU]

Lesion: Any pathological or traumatic discontinuity of tissue or loss of function of a part. [EU]

Listeria: A genus of bacteria which may be found in the feces of animals and man, on vegetation, and in silage. Its species are parasitic on cold-blooded and warm-blooded animals, including man. [NIH]

Lobe: A more or less well-defined portion of any organ, especially of the brain, lungs, and glands. Lobes are demarcated by fissures, sulci, connective tissue, and by their shape. [EU]

Localization: 1. the determination of the site or place of any process or lesion. 2. restriction to a circumscribed or limited area. 3. prelocalization. [EU]

Lupus: A form of cutaneous tuberculosis. It is seen predominantly in women and typically involves the nasal, buccal, and conjunctival mucosa. [NIH]

Lymphadenopathy: Disease of the lymph nodes. [EU]

Lymphoma: Cancer of the lymph nodes. [NIH]

Malignant: Tending to become progressively worse and to result in death. Having the properties of anaplasia, invasion, and metastasis; said of tumours. [EU]

Mediate: Indirect; accomplished by the aid of an intervening medium. [EU]

Mediator: An object or substance by which something is mediated, such as (1) a structure of the nervous system that transmits impulses eliciting a specific response; (2) a chemical substance (transmitter substance) that induces activity in an excitable tissue, such as nerve or muscle; or (3) a substance released from cells as the result of the interaction of antigen with antibody or by the action of antigen with a sensitized lymphocyte. [EU]

Megakaryocytes: Very large bone marrow cells which release mature blood platelets. [NIH]

Membrane: Thin, flexible film of proteins and lipids that encloses the contents of a cell; it controls the substances that go into and come out of the cell. Also, a thin layer of tissue that covers the surface or lines the cavity of an organ. [NIH]

Microbiology: The study of microorganisms such as fungi, bacteria, algae, archaea, and viruses. [NIH]

Microscopy: The application of microscope magnification to the study of materials that cannot be properly seen by the unaided eye. [NIH]

Mobilization: The process of making a fixed part or stored substance mobile, as by separating a part from surrounding structures to make it accessible for an operative procedure or by causing release into the circulation for body use of a substance stored in the body. [EU]

Molecular: Of, pertaining to, or composed of molecules : a very small mass of matter. [EU]

Morphine: The principal alkaloid in opium and the prototype opiate analgesic and narcotic. Morphine has widespread effects in the central nervous system and on smooth muscle. [NIH]

Neoplasms: New abnormal growth of tissue. Malignant neoplasms show a greater degree of anaplasia and have the properties of invasion and metastasis, compared to benign neoplasms. [NIH]

Nephrology: A subspecialty of internal medicine concerned with the anatomy, physiology, and pathology of the kidney. [NIH]

Nephropathy: Disease of the kidneys. [EU]

Nephrotoxic: Toxic or destructive to kidney cells. [EU]

Neural: 1. pertaining to a nerve or to the nerves. 2. situated in the region of the spinal axis, as the neutral arch. [EU]

Neuronal: Pertaining to a neuron or neurons (= conducting cells of the nervous system). [EU]

Neurons: The basic cellular units of nervous tissue. Each neuron consists of a body, an axon, and dendrites. Their purpose is to receive, conduct, and transmit impulses in the nervous system. [NIH]

Niacin: Water-soluble vitamin of the B complex occurring in various animal and plant tissues. Required by the body for the formation of coenzymes NAD and NADP. Has pellagra-curative, vasodilating, and antilipemic properties. [NIH]

Nicotine: Nicotine is highly toxic alkaloid. It is the prototypical agonist at nicotinic cholinergic receptors where it dramatically stimulates neurons and ultimately blocks synaptic transmission. Nicotine is also important medically because of its presence in tobacco smoke. [NIH]

Nosocomial: Pertaining to or originating in the hospital, said of an infection not present or incubating prior to admittance to the hospital, but generally occurring 72 hours after admittance; the term is usually used to refer to patient disease, but hospital personnel may also acquire nosocomial infection. [EU]

Ophthalmology: A surgical specialty concerned with the structure and function of the eye and the medical and surgical treatment of its defects and diseases. [NIH]

Otolaryngology: A surgical specialty concerned with the study and treatment of disorders of the ear, nose, and throat. [NIH]

Overdose: 1. to administer an excessive dose. 2. an excessive dose. [EU]

Overweight: An excess of body weight but not necessarily body fat; a body mass index of 25 to 29.9 kg/m2. [NIH]

Paediatric: Of or relating to the care and medical treatment of children; belonging to or concerned with paediatrics. [EU]

Papillomavirus: A genus of papovaviridae causing proliferation of the epithelium, which may lead to malignancy. A wide range of animals are infected including humans, chimpanzees, cattle, rabbits, dogs, and horses. [NIH]

Paralysis: Loss or impairment of motor function in a part due to lesion of the neural or muscular mechanism; also by analogy, impairment of sensory function (sensory paralysis). In addition to the types named below, paralysis is further distinguished as traumatic, syphilitic, toxic, etc., according to its cause; or as obturator, ulnar, etc., according to the nerve part, or muscle specially affected. [EU]

Pathogenesis: The cellular events and reactions that occur in the development of disease. [NIH]

Pediatrics: A medical specialty concerned with maintaining health and providing medical care to children from birth to adolescence. [NIH]

Pharmacokinetics: The action of drugs in the body over a period of time, including the processes of absorption, distribution, localization in tissues, biotransformation, and excretion. [EU]

Pharmacologic: Pertaining to pharmacology or to the properties and reactions of drugs. [EU]

Phenotype: The entire physical, biochemical, and physiological makeup of an individual as determined by his or her genes and by the environment in the broad sense. [NIH]

Physiologic: Normal; not pathologic; characteristic of or conforming to the normal functioning or state of the body or a tissue or organ; physiological. [EU]

Pigmentation: 1. the deposition of colouring matter; the coloration or discoloration of a part by pigment. 2. coloration, especially abnormally increased coloration, by melanin. [EU]

Plasmapheresis: Procedure whereby plasma is separated and extracted from anticoagulated whole blood and the red cells retransfused to the donor. Plasmapheresis is also employed for therapeutic use. [NIH]

Polypeptide: A peptide which on hydrolysis yields more than two amino acids; called tripeptides, tetrapeptides, etc. according to the number of amino acids contained. [EU]

Postnatal: Occurring after birth, with reference to the newborn. [EU]

Postoperative: Occurring after a surgical operation. [EU]

Potassium: An element that is in the alkali group of metals. It has an atomic symbol K, atomic number 19, and atomic weight 39.10. It is the chief cation in the intracellular fluid of muscle and other cells. Potassium ion is a strong electrolyte and it plays a significant role in the regulation of fluid volume and maintenance of the water-electrolyte balance. [NIH]

Prednisone: A synthetic anti-inflammatory glucocorticoid derived from cortisone. It is biologically inert and converted to prednisolone in the liver. [NIH]

Prophylaxis: The prevention of disease; preventive treatment. [EU]

Proportional: Being in proportion : corresponding in size, degree, or intensity, having the same or a constant ratio; of, relating to, or used in determining proportions. [EU]

Proteins: Polymers of amino acids linked by peptide bonds. The specific sequence of amino acids determines the shape and function of the protein. [NIH]

Psoriasis: A common genetically determined, chronic, inflammatory skin disease characterized by rounded erythematous, dry, scaling patches. The lesions have a predilection for nails, scalp, genitalia, extensor surfaces, and the lumbosacral region. Accelerated epidermopoiesis is considered to be the fundamental pathologic feature in psoriasis. [NIH]

Purpura: Purplish or brownish red discoloration, easily visible through the epidermis, caused by hemorrhage into the tissues. [NIH]

Reactivation: The restoration of activity to something that has been inactivated. [EU]

Receptor: 1. a molecular structure within a cell or on the surface characterized by (1) selective binding of a specific substance and (2) a specific physiologic effect that accompanies the binding, e.g., cell-surface receptors for peptide hormones, neurotransmitters, antigens, complement fragments, and immunoglobulins and cytoplasmic receptors for steroid hormones. 2. a sensory nerve terminal that responds to stimuli of various kinds. [EU]

Recombinant: 1. a cell or an individual with a new combination of genes not found together in either parent; usually applied to linked genes. [EU]

Reconstitution: 1. a type of regeneration in which a new organ forms by the rearrangement of tissues rather than from new formation at an injured surface. 2. the restoration to original form of a substance previously altered for preservation and storage, as the restoration to a liquid state of blood serum or plasma that has been dried and stored. [EU]

Recurrence: The return of a sign, symptom, or disease after a remission. [NIH]

Refractory: Not readily yielding to treatment. [EU]

Remission: A diminution or abatement of the symptoms of a disease; also the period during which such diminution occurs. [EU]

Rheumatoid: Resembling rheumatism. [EU]

Riboflavin: Nutritional factor found in milk, eggs, malted barley, liver, kidney, heart, and leafy vegetables. The richest natural source is yeast. It occurs in the free form only in the retina of the eye, in whey, and in urine; its principal forms in tissues and cells are as FMN and FAD. [NIH]

Salmonella: A genus of gram-negative, facultatively anaerobic, rod-shaped bacteria that utilizes citrate as a sole carbon source. It is pathogenic for humans, causing enteric fevers, gastroenteritis, and bacteremia. Food poisoning is the most common clinical manifestation. Organisms within this genus are separated on the basis of antigenic characteristics, sugar fermentation patterns, and bacteriophage susceptibility. [NIH]

Sarcoma: A tumour made up of a substance like the embryonic connective tissue; tissue composed of closely packed cells embedded in a fibrillar or homogeneous substance. Sarcomas are often highly malignant. [EU]

Sclerosis: A induration, or hardening; especially hardening of a part from inflammation and in diseases of the interstitial substance. The term is used chiefly for such a hardening of the nervous system due to hyperplasia of the connective tissue or to designate hardening of the blood vessels. [EU]

Selenium: An element with the atomic symbol Se, atomic number 34, and atomic weight 78.96. It is an essential micronutrient for mammals and other animals but is toxic in large amounts. Selenium protects intracellular structures against oxidative damage. It is an essential component of glutathione peroxidase. [NIH]

Sepsis: The presence of disease-causing organisms or their toxins in the blood. [NIH]

Serum: The clear portion of any body fluid; the clear fluid moistening serous membranes. 2. blood serum; the clear liquid that separates from blood on clotting. 3. immune serum; blood serum from an immunized animal used for passive immunization; an antiserum; antitoxin, or antivenin. [EU]

Splenomegaly: Enlargement of the spleen. [EU]

Stimulant: 1. producing stimulation; especially producing stimulation by causing tension on muscle fibre through the nervous tissue. 2. an agent or remedy that produces stimulation. [EU]

Stroke: Sudden loss of function of part of the brain because of loss of blood flow. Stroke may be caused by a clot (thrombosis) or rupture (hemorrhage) of a blood vessel to the brain. [NIH]

Subacute: Somewhat acute; between acute and chronic. [EU]

Superinfection: A new infection complicating the course of antimicrobial therapy of an existing infectious process, and resulting from invasion by bacteria or fungi resistant to the drug(s) in use. It may occur at the site of the original infection or at a remote site. [EU]

Suppressive: Tending to suppress : effecting suppression; specifically : serving to suppress activity, function, symptoms. [EU]

Surgical: Of, pertaining to, or correctable by surgery. [EU]

Symptomatic: 1. pertaining to or of the nature of a symptom. 2. indicative (of a particular disease or disorder). 3. exhibiting the symptoms of a particular disease but having a different cause. 4. directed at the allying of symptoms, as symptomatic treatment. [EU]

Synaptic: Pertaining to or affecting a synapse (= site of functional apposition between neurons, at which an impulse is transmitted from one neuron to another by electrical or chemical means); pertaining to synapsis (= pairing off in point-for-point association of homologous chromosomes from the male and female pronuclei during the early prophase of meiosis). [EU]

Synergistic: Acting together; enhancing the effect of another force or agent. [EU]

Systemic: Relating to a process that affects the body generally; in this instance, the way in which blood is supplied through the aorta to all body organs except the lungs. [NIH]

Thalassemia: A group of hereditary hemolytic anemias in which there is decreased synthesis of one or more hemoglobin polypeptide chains. There are several genetic types with clinical pictures ranging from barely detectable hematologic abnormality to severe and fatal anemia. [NIH]

Thermoregulation: Heat regulation. [EU]

Thrombocytopenia: Decrease in the number of blood platelets. [EU]

Thrombosis: The formation, development, or presence of a thrombus. [EU]

Thyroxine: An amino acid of the thyroid gland which exerts a stimulating effect on thyroid metabolism. [NIH]

Tolerance: 1. the ability to endure unusually large doses of a drug or toxin. 2. acquired drug tolerance; a decreasing response to repeated constant doses of a drug or the need for increasing doses to maintain a constant response. [EU]

Toxicity: The quality of being poisonous, especially the degree of virulence of a toxic microbe or of a poison. [EU]

Transfusion: The introduction of whole blood or blood component directly into the blood stream. [EU]

Transplantation: The grafting of tissues taken from the patient's own body or from another. [EU]

Tuberculosis: Any of the infectious diseases of man and other animals caused by species of mycobacterium. [NIH]

Urinary: Pertaining to the urine; containing or secreting urine. [EU]

Uterus: The hollow muscular organ in female mammals in which the fertilized ovum normally becomes embedded and in which the developing embryo and fetus is nourished. In the nongravid human, it is a pear-shaped structure; about 3 inches in length, consisting of a body, fundus, isthmus, and cervix. Its cavity opens into the vagina below, and into the uterine tube on either side at the cornu. It is supported by direct attachment to the vagina and by indirect attachment to various other nearby pelvic structures. Called also metra. [EU]

Vaccination: The introduction of vaccine into the body for the purpose of inducing immunity. Coined originally to apply to the injection of smallpox vaccine, the term has come to mean any immunizing procedure in which vaccine is injected. [EU]

Vaccine: A suspension of attenuated or killed microorganisms (bacteria, viruses, or rickettsiae), administered for the prevention, amelioration or treatment of infectious diseases. [EU]

Varicella: Chicken pox. [EU]

Vascular: Pertaining to blood vessels or indicative of a copious blood supply. [EU]

Vasculitis: Inflammation of a vessel, angiitis. [EU]

Viral: Pertaining to, caused by, or of the nature of virus. [EU]

Viremia: The presence of viruses in the blood. [NIH]

Viruses: Minute infectious agents whose genomes are composed of DNA or RNA, but not both. They are characterized by a lack of independent metabolism and the inability to replicate outside living host cells. [NIH]

Withdrawal: 1. a pathological retreat from interpersonal contact and social involvement, as may occur in schizophrenia, depression, or schizoid avoidant and schizotypal personality disorders. 2. (DSM III-R) a substance-specific organic brain syndrome that follows the cessation of use or reduction in intake of a psychoactive substance that had been regularly used to induce a state of intoxication. [EU]

General Dictionaries and Glossaries

While the above glossary is essentially complete, the dictionaries listed here cover virtually all aspects of medicine, from basic words and phrases to more advanced terms (sorted alphabetically by title; hyperlinks provide rankings, information and reviews at Amazon.com):

- **Dictionary of Medical Acronymns & Abbreviations** by Stanley Jablonski (Editor), Paperback, 4th edition (2001), Lippincott Williams & Wilkins Publishers, ISBN: 1560534605, **http://www.amazon.com/exec/obidos/ASIN/1560534605/icongroupinterna**

- **Dictionary of Medical Terms : For the Nonmedical Person (Dictionary of Medical Terms for the Nonmedical Person, Ed 4)** by Mikel A. Rothenberg, M.D, et al, Paperback - 544 pages, 4th edition (2000), Barrons Educational Series, ISBN: 0764112015, **http://www.amazon.com/exec/obidos/ASIN/0764112015/icongroupinterna**

- **A Dictionary of the History of Medicine** by A. Sebastian, CD-Rom edition (2001), CRC Press-Parthenon Publishers, ISBN: 185070368X, **http://www.amazon.com/exec/obidos/ASIN/185070368X/icongroupinterna**

- **Dorland's Illustrated Medical Dictionary (Standard Version)** by Dorland, et al, Hardcover - 2088 pages, 29th edition (2000), W B Saunders Co, ISBN: 0721662544,
  http://www.amazon.com/exec/obidos/ASIN/0721662544/icongroupinterna

- **Dorland's Electronic Medical Dictionary** by Dorland, et al, Software, 29th Book & CD-Rom edition (2000), Harcourt Health Sciences, ISBN: 0721694934,
  http://www.amazon.com/exec/obidos/ASIN/0721694934/icongroupinterna

- **Dorland's Pocket Medical Dictionary (Dorland's Pocket Medical Dictionary, 26th Ed)** Hardcover - 912 pages, 26th edition (2001), W B Saunders Co, ISBN: 0721682812,
  http://www.amazon.com/exec/obidos/ASIN/0721682812/icongroupinterna
  /103-4193558-7304618

- **Melloni's Illustrated Medical Dictionary (Melloni's Illustrated Medical Dictionary, 4th Ed)** by Melloni, Hardcover, 4th edition (2001), CRC Press-Parthenon Publishers, ISBN: 85070094X,
  http://www.amazon.com/exec/obidos/ASIN/85070094X/icongroupinterna

- **Stedman's Electronic Medical Dictionary Version 5.0 (CD-ROM for Windows and Macintosh, Individual)** by Stedmans, CD-ROM edition (2000), Lippincott Williams & Wilkins Publishers, ISBN: 0781726328,
  http://www.amazon.com/exec/obidos/ASIN/0781726328/icongroupinterna

- **Stedman's Medical Dictionary** by Thomas Lathrop Stedman, Hardcover - 2098 pages, 27th edition (2000), Lippincott, Williams & Wilkins, ISBN: 068340007X,
  http://www.amazon.com/exec/obidos/ASIN/068340007X/icongroupinterna

- **Tabers Cyclopedic Medical Dictionary (Thumb Index)** by Donald Venes (Editor), et al, Hardcover - 2439 pages, 19th edition (2001), F A Davis Co, ISBN: 0803606540,
  http://www.amazon.com/exec/obidos/ASIN/0803606540/icongroupinterna

INDEX

.

Printed in the United States
1345000001B/123-124